REDUCING DIARRHEA IN TUBE-FED PATIENTS

Using Research to Improve Nursing Practice

Other books in this series:

Structured Preoperative Teaching

Preoperative Sensory Preparation to Promote Recovery

Preventing Decubitus Ulcers

Pain: Deliberative Nursing Interventions

Mutual Goal Setting in Patient Care

Closed Urinary Drainage Systems

Clean Intermittent Catheterization

Intravenous Cannula Change

Distress Reduction Through Sensory Preparation

Using Research to Improve Nursing Practice: A Guide

CURN PROJECT STAFF

PRINCIPAL INVESTIGATOR: **Jo Anne Horsley, R.N., Ph.D.**
School of Nursing, The University of Michigan

CO-PRINCIPAL INVESTIGATOR: **Donald C. Pelz, Ph.D.**
Institute for Social Research, The University of Michigan

MNA LIAISON: **Joan S. Guy, R.N., B.S.**
Michigan Nurses Association

RESEARCH UTILIZATION PROGRAM:

Director: Joyce Crane, R.N., M.S.N.
School of Nursing, and Institute for Social Research
The University of Michigan

Research Utilization Training Staff:
D. Jean Wood, R.N., Ph.D., Faculty Associate
School of Nursing, The University of Michigan
Katherine Crabtree, R.N., M.S., Faculty Associate
School of Nursing, Michigan State University
Suzanne Brouse, R.N., M.S., Faculty Associate
School of Nursing, Michigan State University

Protocol Development:
Margaret A. Reynolds, R.N., M.S., Research Associate
School of Nursing, The University of Michigan
Karen B. Haller, R.N., M.S., Research Associate
School of Nursing, The University of Michigan
Janet D. Bingle, R.N., M.S., Faculty Associate
School of Nursing, The University of Michigan

Consultant:
Ronald G. Havelock, Ph.D.
Institute for Social Research, The University of Michigan

COLLABORATIVE RESEARCH PROGRAM:

Director: Maxine E. Loomis, R.N., Ph.D.
School of Nursing, The University of Michigan

Staff:
Kathleen P. Krone, R.N., M.S., Faculty Associate
School of Nursing, The University of Michigan

DATA COLLECTION AND MANAGEMENT:

Data Management:
Laura Klem, A.B., Senior Research Associate
Institute for Social Research, The University of Michigan
Lynn Levin, M.P.H., Research Associate
Institute for Social Research, The University of Michigan
Linda Shepard, B.A., Research Associate
Institute for Social Research, The University of Michigan
Patricia Tomlin, M.A., Research Associate
Institute for Social Research, The University of Michigan

Research Assistants:
Jane Anderson, R.N., M.S., Data Analysis
School of Nursing, The University of Michigan
Mary Best, R.N., M.S., Data Editor
School of Nursing, The University of Michigan
Judith Fry, R.N., M.S., Data Collection
School of Nursing, The University of Michigan
Cheryl White, R.N., M.S., Data Collection
School of Nursing, The University of Michigan

SUPPORT STAFF:

Editor:
Vivian Collier, M.Ed.
School of Nursing, The University of Michigan

Principal Secretary:
Margaret Horn
Institute for Social Research, The University of Michigan

Administrative Assistants:
Kathryn Horne, A.B.
School of Nursing, The University of Michigan
Barbara Welmers
Michigan Nurses Association

REDUCING DIARRHEA IN TUBE-FED PATIENTS

CURN Project

Conduct and Utilization of Research in Nursing Project
Michigan Nurses Association

Principal Investigator:
Jo Anne Horsley, R.N., Ph.D.

This book is a product of the Research Utilization Program, CURN Project.
Director:
Joyce Crane, R.N., M.S.N.

The protocol manuscript for this book was prepared by:
Karen B. Haller, R.N., M.S.

This project was supported by the Division of Nursing, DHEW, Grant RO2 NU00542, and conducted under the auspices of the Michigan Nurses Association. The scientific work of the Project was conducted at The University of Michigan School of Nursing and Institute for Social Research and at Michigan State University School of Nursing.

Grune & Stratton

A Subsidiary of Harcourt Brace Jovanovich, Publishers
New York London Toronto Sydney San Francisco

Grune & Stratton, Inc.
111 Fifth Avenue
New York, New York 10003

Distributed in the United Kingdom by
Academic Press Inc. (London) Ltd.
24/28 Oval Road, London NW 1

Library of Congress Catalog Number 81-1419
International Standard Book Number 0-8089-1326-3

Printed in the United States of America

CONTENTS

ACKNOWLEDGMENTS

The work of the CURN Project could not have been completed without the participation of nursing departments in hospitals throughout the State of Michigan. In all, thirty-four nursing departments worked with the CURN Project staff in the following capacities: Research Utilization Program intervention (experimental) sites, Research Utilization Program comparison sites, and Collaborative Research Program sites.

Research Utilization Program: Intervention (Experimental) Sites

Detroit Memorial Hospital (Detroit–Macomb Hospitals Association), Detroit

Genesee Memorial Hospital, Flint
Grace Hospital Division (Harper–Grace Hospitals), Detroit
Harper Hospital Division (Harper–Grace Hospitals), Detroit
Henry Ford Hospital, Detroit
Hurley Medical Center, Flint
Lapeer County General Hospital, Lapeer
McLaren General Hospital, Flint
Metropolitan Hospital (Metropolitan Hospital and Health Center), Detroit
Midland Hospital Center, Midland
Mount Carmel Mercy Hospital, Detroit
Providence Hospital, Southfield
Rehabilitation Institute, Detroit
Saginaw Community Hospital, Saginaw
St. Joseph Mercy Hospital (Samaritan Health Center), Detroit
Sinai Hospital of Detroit, Detroit
South Macomb Hospital (Detroit–Macomb Hospitals Association), Detroit

Research Utilization Program: Comparison Sites

Emma L. Bixby Hospital, Adrian
Bon Secours Hospital, Grosse Pointe
Chelsea Community Hospital, Chelsea
Community Health Center of Branch County, Coldwater
Cottage Hospital of Grosse Pointe, Grosse Pointe Farms
W.A. Foote Memorial Hospital, Jackson
Holy Cross Hospital, Detroit
McPherson Community Health Center, Howell
Mercy–Memorial Hospital, Monroe
North Detroit General Hospital, Detroit
St. John Hospital, Detroit
St. Joseph Mercy Hospital (Catherine McAuley Health Center) Ann Arbor
Southwest Detroit Hospital, Detroit
Veterans Administration Medical Center, Allen Park
Veterans Administration Medical Center, Ann Arbor

Collaborative Research Program Sites

Bon Secours Hospital, Grosse Pointe
Children's Hospital of Michigan, Detroit
Henry Ford Hospital, Detroit
Little Traverse Hospital (Northern Michigan Hospitals), Petoskey
McLaren General Hospital, Flint
Rehabilitation Institute, Detroit

PREFACE

The body of scientific knowledge on which the practice of nursing rests is ever increasing. As a natural consequence, there is a growing urgency within the profession to have that knowledge become the basis for delivery of nursing care. This book represents one of the outcomes of a research project designed to develop and test a model to facilitate the use of scientific nursing knowledge in clinical practice settings. In this book, scientific nursing knowledge is defined as knowledge that has been generated by research studies that used various methods of modern science to investigate nursing problems. The outcomes of these investigations include not only the research results, but also the scientific methods and technology used by investigators while conducting their studies.

One of the major barriers to the clinical utilization of scientific nursing knowledge arises from the varied contexts in which nurse clinicians and nurse scientists work. Differences in the goals and methods employed by each are of primary importance. For example, nursing care is generally conceived of as individualized care; that is, patients receive care based on their unique needs and attributes (and the nurse's unique knowledge and skills). The focus is on individual differences as they occur in both patients and nurses. The nurse scientist, while cognizant of individual differences, seeks to identify and control phenomena, e.g., nursing interventions and patient outcomes, that are applicable to identifiable groups of patients and nurses. The scientist tries to minimize the impact of individual differences. In order to produce a science of nursing practice, nurse clinicians and nurse scientists must recognize and appreciate this type of variance in each other's goals and methods and perform their respective activities from a stance of mutual respect and identification.

This book represents one attempt to move research and practice closer together by transforming research outcomes into useful clinical knowledge that can be scientifically implemented in practice settings. Research studies are not, ipso facto, scientifically sound or clinically useful. Their scientific merit and clinical utility should be ascertained before clinical practice implementation is attempted. Three sets of criteria were used to screen the research on lactose-free tube-feeding diets before it was transformed into the clinical protocol in this book. The research studies were reviewed to (1) determine the validity and reliability of the knowledge they generated; (2) determine the relevance of the knowledge for clinical practice settings; and (3) determine the availability of evaluation instruments necessary to measure the effectiveness of subsequent clinical practice changes. This screening process was used to identify research that both embodied goals and used methods applicable to clinical practice.

When scientifically sound and clinically useful research has been identified, a clinical protocol can then be developed. The purpose of a clinical protocol is to transform the knowledge, methods, and technology inherent in the research studies into knowledge, methods, and technology useful to clinicians. The protocol carefully maintains the scientific integrity of the original research. Once the protocol is developed, it becomes the user's responsibility to understand and appreciate the work of the scientists who produced the knowledge base.

The book is designed to help users—be they clinicians, teachers, or students—understand and appreciate the knowledge base that supports lactose-free tube-feeding formulas. Chapter 1 contains a general introduction to the protocol, orienting the user to its various components and the parts they play in clinical implementation. Chapter 2 contains the entire protocol, which synthesizes and transforms the research into clinically useful knowledge. It also presents a section on clinical evaluation, which is required in order to determine whether the integrity of the original research has been maintained in the practice change. In Chapter 3 are reprints of selected research articles that have a primary function in relation to the protocol. It is necessary to review each of these articles to develop an understanding of the knowledge base and enhance awareness of technological advances necessary for sound clinical implementation. A guide to assist the reader with the research article review is included in Appendix A.

A clinical protocol, regardless of its inherent quality, cannot guard against misuse that arises from faulty implementation processes. Scientific knowledge is relatively precise. It deserves, in fact, dictates, a scientific approach to its use in practice. A handbook, **Using Research To Improve Nursing Practice: A Guide**, has been written to help users learn the tasks involved in producing practice change that maintains the scientific integrity of a knowledge base and minimizes disruption to the ongoing activities of the department of nursing. The reader of this volume and any other clinical protocol is strongly urged to use the handbook as a guide for practice change activities.

Many people have contributed to the project that spawned this book. Special mention is indicated for some without whose vision and active support the project might never have happened.

The Council for Nursing Research of the Michigan Nurses Association (MNA) laid the groundwork for the project when it adopted "closing the gap between research and practice" as one of its primary goals. The project was carried out under the auspices of the MNA, and we thank the MNA Board of Directors, the Council for Nursing Research, and especially Mrs. Joan S. Guy for their courage in taking up the challenge to close the research–practice gap.

Thirty-two nursing departments participated in the Research Utilization Program of the CURN Project. The directors of these departments and their respective staff members actively shaped the protocols and utilization process in the hope that they would be useful for themselves, their clinical colleagues, and the profession.

The "Regional Program for Nursing Research and Development" project, carried out by staff members from the Western Interstate Commission for Higher Education (WICHE), preceded our work in research utilization. Three members of the staff of that project deserve mention because of their tireless efforts to share the outcomes of their work in hopes that it would further our work. Janelle Krueger and Carol Lindeman, Principal Investigators of the project, and Jo Eleanor Elliott, Director of WCHEN, demonstrated the true spirit of sharing knowledge and offering colleague support.

We want to acknowledge the many scientists without whose research there would be no scientific knowledge to use in practice. We are especially grateful to those whose work served as the basis for this protocol.

For the past five years, ten nurses have served as members of the CURN Project Advisory Committee: Amy Barbus, Mary Castles, Joan Guy, Barbara Horn, Ada Jacox, Corinne Bachle Kordyson, Carol Lindeman, Sally Lechlitner Lusk, Dorothea Milbrandt, and Carolyn Williams. They served us well over the years—questioning, offering advice, giving support, always encouraging, and expecting the best but never the impossible.

Doris Bloch, Chief of the Research Grants Section, Nursing Research Branch of the Division of Nursing, DHEW, has served as our project officer. Her vision of the intimate and interdependent relationship between research and practice was apparent from the earliest conception of the project, and over the years she has served as a positive stimulus for our work. Further, her faith in a young, naive research staff never appeared to waver; it sustained us when our faith sometimes failed.

We also want to acknowledge the work of the many staff members who learned, worked, created, enjoyed, and at times despaired as the project moved forward. Of special note are: Margaret Reynolds, Karen Haller, and Janet Bingle, who were responsible for the preparation of the clinical protocols; the "linkers," D. Jean Wood, Katherine Crabtree, and Suzanne Brouse, who provided valuable insights regarding the clinical implementation of the protocols; and Ronald Havelock, who provided the basic model on which the work was based. We especially wish to thank Vivian Collier and Kathryn Horne, who somehow endured the unending detail involved in the preparation of this manuscript.

Donald Pelz was the Co-Principal Investigator for the project. Throughout the five years we worked together, he was a steady influence, bringing his knowledge and experience in the field of knowledge utilization to bear on the field of nursing. While never claiming to be an expert on nursing, he respected and sought to understand the aspects of our field that influence the process of research utilization. We thank him for his willingness to share of himself and to be open to others.

Jo Anne Horsley
Principal Investigator
CURN Project

Joyce Crane
Program Director
Research Utilization Program

Chapter 1
INTRODUCTION: USING RESEARCH TO IMPROVE NURSING PRACTICE

Over the past three decades, the nursing profession has experienced a steady increase in research activity and growth in production of research-based knowledge. Yet application of the knowledge to practice has been slow to occur. Of necessity, nursing practice consists largely of "stereotyped techniques sprinkled liberally with personal idiosyncracy" (Lysaught, 1970, p. 84).

RESEARCH-BASED NURSING KNOWLEDGE

The identification of scientific knowledge for use in practice begins with the retrieval and review of studies. Studies which contribute to a single area of research form a "base" from which nursing knowledge may be derived. When the activities suggested by the research base are different from traditional practice—that is, either add to practice in some way or call for the extinction of a practice—they constitute an "innovation." Innovations in nursing imply changes in practice that are new to those using them. These innovations may include a change in a nursing intervention, a method of evaluation, or a means for producing clinical data.

Certainly not all research is ready to be applied in the practice setting; in fact, premature utilization of research findings may prove harmful. To identify research that *is* ready for use in practice, specific criteria have been developed and organized into three major categories (Haller, Reynolds, & Horsley, 1979; reprinted in the Appendix).

The first category concerns the evaluation of related studies that comprise a conceptual base. These criteria include: (1) the need for replication to provide greater confidence in the reliability and validity of findings; (2) examination of each study's scientific merit, especially concerning validity, reliability, generality, and statistical significance; and (3) determination of any potential risk to patients.

The second category concerns the relevance of the scientific knowledge to practice or the extent to which it addresses a nursing problem in a clinical setting. At issue here are such factors as clinical merit or significance, the extent to which practicing nurses have clinical control over the independent and dependent variables, the feasibility of implementation, and the cost of implementation weighed against the expected benefits.

The final category concerns the potential for clinical evaluation of the practice change. To assure a purposeful evaluation, there must be at least one dependent variable in the research base, and preferably more, which can be reliably measured by clinicians in practice settings. In other words, clinicians must have the skill required for measurement, and they must have access to reliable measurement tools.

Research-based nursing practice offers specific advantages over traditional practice. Because research is structured and the variables are defined, the knowledge produced is more useful in guiding and evaluating practice: interventions can be defined and outcomes predicted using research-based knowledge. Research also clarifies the limits of knowledge; for example, it specifies the client groups for whom an intervention is likely to be beneficial.

THE RESEARCH-BASED INNOVATION PROTOCOL

Rarely is new knowledge produced in a form that can be directly translated into principles for practice or nursing actions. To be useful, the knowledge must be transformed; that is, it must be converted into a form that can be readily used by practitioners. The "protocol" is a transformation of research-based knowledge. Its purpose is to organize research concerning specific nursing care problems in such a way that the knowledge can be used to direct nursing practice activities. Therefore, the content of the protocol is directed toward implementation and evaluation of the practice change.

Each protocol begins with a section on the need for change. This introductory material documents the extent of the clinical problem and the relevance of the problem to nursing practice. The second section gives a description of the innovation, including information on the types of patients who would be likely to benefit from it. Next, the protocol provides a summary of the research base. The summary is not intended to be a comprehensive review of the literature, but to present a synopsis of the findings which supported the innovation at the time the review was done. Limitations of the research base are also discussed.

In each protocol, a research-based principle is identified to guide the innovation.[1] The remainder of the protocol deals with implementation of the innovation and evaluation of its effects. Selection of an appropriate patient population, the materials that will be required, and the personnel development that will be necessary are discussed in detail. Supplementary material is appended to the protocol where it may be useful to practitioners. These materials may include a selected, annotated bibliography, a sample evaluation procedure, and any additional tools or resources that are available from the original researchers or from others who have utilized the research findings.

---

[1]Although the use of the term "principle" is not scientifically accurate, it has been found to communicate the appropriate intent to most nurses who have used protocols. It is more accurate, however, to say that what is derived from a research base is an "empirical generalization."

USING A PROTOCOL

Protocols are designed to be used in conjunction with published studies from the research base, a reading guide, and a process handbook. The protocol is not intended to be read in lieu of the original research. For convenience, the studies to be read in conjunction with the protocol have been reprinted in Chapter 3. It is suggested that the protocol be read prior to reviewing the studies; then, having read the original research, it will be useful to read the protocol again.

A tool to assist practitioners to critically review the research literature has been reprinted in the Appendix. This tool, *Guide to Reading Research Critically,* was designed for use in reviewing and understanding the major studies which address a practice problem. The guide is organized as a series of questions to help nurses identify what has been tested, with what population, under what circumstances, using which techniques or tools.

The handbook, *Using Research to Improve Nursing Practice: A Guide,* is designed to assist clinicians to carry out practice changes in a way that maintains the scientific integrity of the original research. For example, the handbook describes a process that (1) assures a practice activity will adequately represent the intervention suggested by the research base and (2) generates data to demonstrate the effectiveness of the change. When an innovation is to be implemented in a clinical setting, it is essential that the handbook be used in conjunction with the protocol. The handbook describes one complete sequence of activities necessary to accomplish research-based change in nursing practice, while the protocol provides specific information about an innovation. The use of the protocol with the handbook will guide practitioners in conducting a successful trial of the innovation.

Chapter 2
CLINICAL PROTOCOL: REDUCING DIARRHEA IN TUBE-FED PATIENTS

THE NEED FOR CHANGE

Tube feeding has been defined as "The administration of a complete, nutritionally adequate liquid diet by means of a tube passing into the stomach. The tube may be inserted through the nose or mouth and esophagus or through a surgically formed fistula directly into the esophagus (esophagostomy) or stomach (gastrostomy)" (Walike, 1976). Tube feeding is a common procedure whose simplicity belies the complications frequently associated with it.

Walike, et al. (1975) surveyed 121 patients to assess practices and problems associated with tube feedings. Most of the data were collected retrospectively from patient charts; however, 41 patients were also hospitalized during data collection. Changes in stool frequency and consistency were among the most frequently recorded responses to nasogastric tube feeding. The data revealed that 14 percent of the patients had three or more stools per day for the 20-day study period. Data also revealed generally diarrhea-like stools: "more watery to soft-formed stools were reported than normal to dry stools"(Hanson, et al., 1975). Other reports of the incidence of diarrhea associated with tube feeding have ranged from 7 percent (Pareira, 1959) to 20 percent (Jones and Peaston, 1966).

Diarrhea associated with tube feeding has been causally linked to the use of milk-based formulas (Walike and Walike, 1973, 1977). This diarrhea has been explained by the researchers as a result of a *relative* deficiency of the enzyme lactase in many adults.[1] It follows that adults who are relatively deficient in lactase are also relatively intolerant of lactose, which is the primary sugar in milk; they are thus less able to digest and absorb lactose.

> Lactase is required to split the disaccharide, lactose, into its component monosaccharides, glucose and galactose, which are absorbed in the small intestine. With lactase deficiency, the unsplit lactose passes into the large intestine where it apparently acts by two methods to produce diarrhea. It exerts an osmotic force in the colon, thus drawing fluids into the lumen, and the lactose is fermented by bacteria into organic acids which act as irritants to the mucosa of the large intestine. The results are cramping, gas production, borborygmi, and diarrhea. (Walike and Walike, 1973)

It has been noted that findings such as these "raise considerable question when one considers that most house-formula or commercial tube-feeding diets have a milk base" (Hanson et al., 1975).

It has been suggested (Walike and Walike, 1973) that diarrhea associated with tube feeding can "cause or contribute to excoriation, discomfort, and generally retarded postoperative progress." It

[1]*In contrast to classical lactose intolerance, relative lactose intolerance is not detected by a lactose tolerance test and only produces clinical symptoms when a large quantity of lactose is ingested. Data have been presented (Walike and Walike, 1973) to support the contention that many who have a relative intolerance to lactose also have a deficiency of lactase, which results in "a delayed and probably incomplete splitting of lactose." Walike and Walike (1977) considered lactose intolerance to be a "relative phenomenon that must be defined by both the size of the lactose load and the total intestinal capacity to hydrolyze lactose."*

has also been shown (Walike, 1969) that the severe complication of "tube-feeding syndrome," which involves dehydration, hypernatremia, hyperchloremia, and azotemia, may be initiated or exacerbated by diarrhea.

DESCRIPTION OF THE INNOVATION

The innovation suggested by the research base is the elimination of lactose from the formulas of tube-feeding diets for adult patients in order to minimize diarrhea, distention, flatulence, fullness, and to reduce patient rejection of feedings. Since lactose is the primary sugar in milk, this innovation calls for the elimination of milk-based formulas and suggests their replacement with commercially prepared lactose-free diets or hospital-formulated meat/vegetable-based diets.

Adult patients with a lactase deficiency who are receiving tube feedings may be expected to benefit from the innovation. The prevalence of lactase deficiency is known to vary by racial group. Proportionately, a greater benefit can be expected among nonwhites. Welsh (1970) reported that lactase deficiency has been demonstrated in 60–70 percent of black Americans and 6–20 percent of white Americans. In reviewing similar data, Walike and Walike (1973) commented as follows:

> One might at this point conclude that lactose-free diets should be used for non-Caucasian patients, but that among Caucasians this would not be so important, due to the small percentage of intolerant adults. Clinically, however, it was our impression that diarrhea occurred in more than 5–10 percent of our Caucasian patients.

Since lactose is not necessary for adequate nutrition, its elimination from the tube-feeding diets of all adult patients is deemed safe. When all patients are considered collectively, the elimination of lactose from tube-feeding diets can be expected to result in "more comfortable and efficient" tube feeding (Walike and Walike, 1973).

SUMMARY OF THE RESEARCH BASE

This protocol is based largely on two clinical studies done by Walike and Walike (1973, 1977). These studies demonstrate that the elimination of lactose from tube-feeding diets can reduce gastrointestinal side effects.

The first study tested two diets, differing in the presence or absence of lactose.[2] Both diets were otherwise identical except for an increased amount of corn syrup solids in the lactose-free diet to make it equivalent in caloric value to the lactose-containing diet. The study population consisted of 11 patients who had head and neck malignancies but who were in general good health with no history of gastrointestinal, renal, neurological, or endocrine disorders. Both diets were administered to each patient in a double-blind fashion:

> Patients were placed on each of the two tube feeding diets for 10 consecutive days. One-half of the group received the lactose diet first, then the non-lactose diet; the other half were given the diets in the reverse order. The order of the diets for each patient was not known to either the physician or nurses involved in the patient care and data collection. The amount of intake was determined by the needs of each patient. (Walike and Walike, 1973).

The same study found that both stool frequency and stool consistency differed between the two diet periods. Stool frequency was two to four times greater on the lactose-containing diet. A comparison of stool consistency between diet periods indicated that the stools were looser and more liquid when patients were on the lactose-containing diet.

In the second study (Walike and Walike, 1977), the researchers replicated their findings with a sample of 16 white adult patients who were receiving nasogastric tube feedings after surgery for head or neck carcinomas. None of these patients had a previous history of intolerance to milk.

Each of the two liquid diets, differing only in the presence or absence of lactose, was administered to each patient for 4 to 9 consecutive days per diet. Both diets contained all the required nutrients, vitamins, and minerals; in addition, they both had a caloric density of 1 kcal per cc. The liquid diet was administered at 2000–3000 kcal per day, six feedings per day.

Although caloric intake did not differ much between the two diets, most patients had at least 1.5 times as many stools on the lactose-containing diet. Stool consistency was predominantly loose

---

[2] *ENSURE ™ by Ross Laboratories.*

to liquid when receiving the 7 percent lactose diet, but it ranged from soft to hard on the lactose-free diet. In addition, Walike and Walike (1977) found that most patients experienced more than one symptom while receiving the lactose diet: "During the lactose diet period, nine patients complained of gastrointestinal distress, including flatulence, borborygmi, belching, nausea, and distention." On the basis of their work then, the researchers recommended the elimination of lactose from the formulas of liquid diets "to minimize diarrhea, distention, flatulence, fullness, and rejection of tube-feeding amounts needed for adequate intake."

RESEARCH-BASED PRINCIPLE TO GUIDE THE INNOVATION

A relative lactose intolerance—that is, an inability to completely digest and absorb lactose—occurs in a substantial percentage of the adult population. Lactase deficiency becomes clinically significant when intolerant patients are fed the relatively large amounts of lactose which are present in milk-based liquid diets. In lactose-intolerant individuals, unabsorbed lactose enters the ileum and colon, producing the symptoms of diarrhea, distention, borborygmus, and flatulence.

Elimination of lactose from the formulas of liquid diets has been shown to reduce gastrointestinal side effects. This effect has been demonstrated on adult patients who were being tube-fed. Elimination of lactose might also benefit other adult patients who ingest large quantities of milk, for example, those on full liquid diets, ulcer patients, and pregnant women; however, the effect of lactose elimination has not been tested in these populations.

IMPLEMENTATION OF THE INNOVATION

The innovation can be implemented on any unit where adult patients receive nasogastric tube feedings. This section will specify the materials required for implementation, as well as the personnel development that will be necessary.

Materials Required

Implementation of the innovation calls for the elimination of milk-based (lactose-containing) tube-feeding diets in favor of lactose-free diets. Either commercially prepared or hospital-formulated lactose-free diets may be used. The lactose-free diet is the only new material required to implement this innovation with any given patient. Generally, all tube-feeding patients may be placed on a lactose-free diet; however, the diet must also be tailored to the specific nutritional needs of the individual patient. For example, some patients may need low-sodium diets, low-residue diets, elemental diets, or low-protein diets. A range of lactose-free diets, therefore, needs to be available to implement the innovation appropriately.

Personnel Development

Implementation of a successful trial is likely to depend on the development of working relationships with other health professionals. If physicians are responsible for ordering the diet, for example, their cooperation will be essential. The dietetics department may be instrumental in ordering or formulating diets. In some institutions, the pharmacy may order and dispense tube-feeding formulas made by commercial laboratories. Involvement of other professionals at an early stage in planning the implementation of this innovation will be essential.

KNOWLEDGE. To successfully implement the innovation, all staff (nursing and nonnursing) who will be involved with the change in tube-feeding diet and/or with tube-fed patients should be included in staff development efforts. Staff development should include a complete description of the innovation, its objectives, and the expected benefits. Understanding of the innovation will require knowledge about: (1) the prevalence of lactose intolerance, (2) the clinical significance of relative lactose intolerance, and (3) the physiologic mechanisms whereby lactose produces gastrointestinal symptoms in lactose-intolerant individuals.

PRACTICE SKILLS. No new practice skills are necessary for implementation of the innovation.

EVALUATION OF THE EFFECTS OF THE INNOVATION

Sample Selection

The effect of the innovation has been demonstrated on adult patients receiving nasogastric tube feedings. A comparable sample should be selected for the trial. Since not all hospitals will have a sizable population of tube-fed patients, it is advisable to gather preliminary data to determine the number of these patients present in a specific institution before proceeding with a trial of the innovation. As a guideline, a minimum of 10 patients should be on nasogastric tube feedings within a period of time acceptable for baseline (or postimplementation) data collection. The patients should also be likely to remain on tube-feeding diets for 7 days or longer to ensure ample time for evaluation.

In addition to the problem of securing an adequate sample, the location of patients within the physical plant may be problematic. It is unlikely that all patients on tube feedings will be located on a single unit. Therefore, for purposes of the trial, it may be necessary to: (1) relocate patients to a trial unit, (2) implement the innovation on a unit with a high proportion of tube-feeding patients, or (3) devise a system to identify and follow patients throughout the hospital.

Evaluation Design

Evaluation of the change to lactose-free tube-feeding diets is designed in three parts: (1) a baseline data collection, (2) implementation of the innovation, and (3) postimplementation data collection. Figure 1 illustrates this sequence. Evaluation of the effects of the innovation is done by comparing the baseline data with the postimplementation data. In planning to make such comparisons, however, consideration should be given to selecting similar types of patients for the two groups (baseline and postimplementation); this will allow a more valid comparison. Although it is not necessary

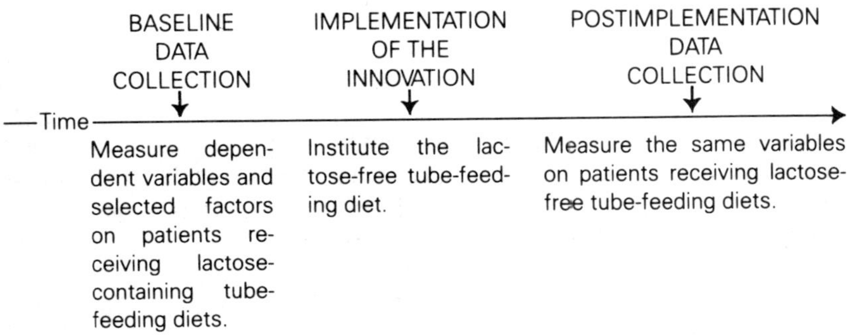

Fig. 1. **Evaluation design: Reducing diarrhea in tube-fed patients.**

to match the groups, there should be reasonable certainty that they are comparable on relevant factors. In this protocol, it is desirable that the two groups be similar on such factors as age, race or ethnic background, and diagnosis.

Variable Selection

Two dependent variables have been found that demonstrate the benefit of the lactose-free diet most clearly. These are *stool frequency* and *stool consistency;* both variables should be measured to evaluate the effects of the innovation. The following describes these two dependent variables, as well as others which may be used in the evaluation design.

STOOL FREQUENCY. Each occurrence of a stool should be recorded for every patient in the baseline and postimplementation groups. The total number of occurrences in a 24-hour period constitutes the measure of stool frequency.

STOOL CONSISTENCY. A stool-consistency rating should be done for each occurrence of a stool. Stool consistency can be rated using the following scale developed by Walike and associates.

1 = Watery
2 = Liquid, creamy
3 = Very loose, mushy, semiliquid
4 = Loose, soft
5 = Formed with some liquid
6 = Soft, formed
7 = Normal, formed
8 = Hard
9 = Hard, dry

Walike and Walike (1977) demonstrated that stool ratings done by nurse clinicians, using this scale in conjunction with stool-consistency diagrams, can be validated by stool-ash analyses.[3] Thus, stool-consistency diagrams with an accompanying scale (see Sup-

[3] *Stool ash is the residue remaining after burning off the combustible components of the stool.*

plement B) can be expected to be useful for evaluation in the clinical setting if used reliably. Interrater reliability will need to be established on the use of the stool-consistency tool prior to the trial of the innovation (see pp. 14–16 for a discussion of interrater reliability). Laboratory analyses, then, will not be necessary for adequate evaluation.

OTHER EVALUATIVE MEASURES. In addition to the two major dependent variables in the research base, it is desirable to measure other potential effects of the innovation. For example, Walike and Walike (1977) noted that many tube-fed patients complain of gastrointestinal distress while on the lactose-containing diet. It is possible to monitor the occurrence of variables which indicate gastrointestinal distress; these include nausea, burping or belching, borborygmi, flatulence, and distention. Another variable of possible interest to clinicians is the amount of tube feeding which is not tolerated—that is, vomited or refused—on each diet.

INFLUENCING FACTORS. Consideration should be given to collecting data about variables which may influence the results achieved. For example, some medications may alter stool consistency and frequency; among these are iron, antacids, and antibiotics, as well as laxatives and antidiarrhetics. Data on clients' stool histories (average number of stools per day and usual stool consistency) may also be useful in interpreting the results of the trial.

Materials Needed

In order to evaluate the effect of the innovation, no equipment will be required that is not already available on patient-care units. It will be necessary, however, to have some forms or flow sheets on which to collect and compile the trial data. Examples of evaluation forms are shown in Supplement C.

Personnel Development

It is essential that evaluation of the innovation is planned well and carried out consistently. Therefore, a staff development program is needed to address the process of evaluation, its purpose and importance, as well as the methods employed to conduct a systematic evaluation. All personnel who will be involved in evaluation need to be aware of the overall plan for carrying out this process.

Nurses who will be using the stool-consistency diagrams and rating scale will need some additional training. It is important that nurses using this measurement tool *independently* can arrive at the same consistency rating when assessing the same specimen. The degree to which agreement between raters can be achieved is called "interrater reliability."

Training activities should be designed to develop reliability in the use of the stool-consistency tool. First, orientation to the diagrams and scale will help to provide a common understanding of the tool, promoting such reliability. Second, nurses who will be doing ratings will need to practice this skill. It will be most useful for these nurses to do a number of ratings on a range of stool consistencies—that is, practice ratings should not all be done on "normal" stools. It will be helpful to practice in pairs, compare individual ratings, and discuss instances of disagreement. It is best for any nurse–rater to rotate with as many partners as possible; in this manner, each rater will have an opportunity to compare results with every other rater and work toward overall agreement.

For purposes of establishing interrater reliability here, perfect agreement between raters is probably not necessary. Agreement may be defined as no more than a one-point difference on the stool-consistency scale between raters. Conversely, disagreement may be defined as a difference greater than one point between raters.

After the training period, interrater reliability should be determined before proceeding with baseline evaluation. For this purpose, all nurse–raters should do a stool-consistency rating in tandem with all other nurse–raters. Although the ratings made by each member of the rater pair will need to be done at the same time on the same specimen, they should be done independently. Figure 2 shows a sample system where two nurses from each shift are assigned to do ratings; each nurse is paired with every other nurse on the grid. For example, RN_3 works on the evening shift; she is paired on the grid with RN_4, who also works the evening shift, as well as with RN_1, RN_2, RN_5, and RN_6, who work other shifts. Thus, RN_3 is a member of five rater pairs and is most often teamed with a nurse from a different shift. Since each member of a rater pair must rate the same specimen at the same time, this will probably best be done at shift change when both members are

		RN_1	RN_2	RN_3	RN_4	RN_5	RN_6
Day Shift	RN_1						
	RN_2	A					
Evening Shift	RN_3	D	A				
	RN_4	A	A	D			
Night Shift	RN_5	A	A	A	A		
	RN_6	A	A	A	A	A	

Fig. 2. Interrater reliability: Sample grid. (A = Agreement; D = Disagreement.)

on duty. It should be noted that all pairs do not rate the same specimen; that is, the 15 ratings represented in Figure 2 involve 15 rater pairs and 15 specimens.[4] Agreement is indicated by an **A,** and disagreement, by a **D**.

Interrater reliability may be calculated as follows, and is expressed as a percentage:

$$\text{Interrater reliability} = \frac{\text{Number of agreements (A)}}{\text{Number of ratings (N)}} \times 100 = \_\_\_\_\_\_\_ \text{ percent}$$

For example, with the sample data shown in Figure 2, an interrater reliability of 86.67 percent would be achieved:

$$\frac{A}{N} \times 100 = \frac{13}{15} \times 100 = 86.67 \text{ percent}$$

An interrater reliability of 80 percent is considered sufficient for purposes of evaluation here. Low interrater reliability may suggest a need for further training. For instance, one or two raters may have reduced the overall reliability, and these individuals may need additional practice. It is also possible that all raters may have diffi-

[4]*If each rater pair had done two ratings, the grid would be completely filled, and the total number of ratings would be 30. Fifteen ratings may be taken as the minimum to be done.*

culty with a certain section of the scale. In the latter case, clearer decision rules for scoring specimens may be needed. After additional training, interrater reliability should be determined again using a new set of ratings. Once acceptable interrater reliability has been achieved, it is important that nurses continue to use the tool exactly as they were trained. Otherwise, interrater reliability will be reduced when the tool is employed in actual data collections.

SUMMARY

The lactose-free tube-feeding protocol has not been piloted yet in a clinical site. The hospitals which have considered the use of it have had tube-feeding patients who were experiencing diarrhea; however, at those hospitals it was determined that the use of lactose-free formulas had already been instituted. It should be noted that the innovation suggested by the research base will not reduce the incidence of diarrhea due to causes other than lactose-containing diets, for example, from contamination or spoilage of the formula.

For those hopsitals where the change suggested by the research base has not been implemented, a reduction in the incidence of diarrhea following implementation of the innovation can be expected. The research base also suggests that a reduction in other symptoms of gastrointestinal distress may be achieved; these include nausea, belching, borborygmi, flatulence, and distention.

It can be postulated that if elimination of lactose from the diet can bring about a reduction in diarrhea and other gastrointestinal symptoms, then some additional benefits might also accrue to tube-fed patients. For example, a reduction in patient discomfort might occur as a result of reduced symptoms; fewer instances of excoriation might result from fewer patients with diarrhea. Although not explicitly demonstrated in the research base, it is possible that tube feeding might become more effective as a result of fewer patient refusals of feedings, allowing a greater caloric intake overall. It has also been suggested that a lactose-associated diarrhea may cause a loss of nutrients in the feces; therefore, a reduction in stool frequency and an improvement in stool consistency might have a postive nutritional effect. These potential benefits need further study in research settings.

REFERENCES

Hanson, R. L., Walike, B. C., Grant, M., Kubo, W., Bergstrom, N., Padilla, G., & Wong, H. L. Patient responses and problems associated with tube feeding. *Washington State Journal of Nursing,* Winter 1975, 9–13.

Jones, E. S., & Peaston, M.J.T. Metabolic care during acute illnesses. *The Practitioner,* 1966, *196,* 271–275.

Pareira, M. D. *Therapeutic nutrition with tube feeding.* Springfield, Ill.: Chas C Thomas, 1959.

Walike, B. C. Disturbances of food intake and nutrition. In H. Moidel, B. Wagner, and E. Giblin (Eds.), *Nursing care of the patient with medical–surgical disorders* (2nd ed.). New York: McGraw-Hill Co., 1976.

*Walike, B. C., Padilla, G., Bergstrom, N., Hanson, R. L., Kubo, W., Grant, M., & Wong, H. L. Patient problems related to tube feeding. In M. V. Batey (Ed.), *Communicating Nursing Research* (vol. 7). Boulder, Colo.: WICHE, 1975.

*Walike, B. C., & Walike, J. W. Lactose content of tube feeding diets as a cause of diarrhea. *The Laryngoscope,* 1973, *83,* 1109–1115.

*Walike, B. C., & Walike, J. W. Relative lactose intolerance. *Journal of the American Medical Association,* 1977, *238,* 948–951.

Walike, J. W. Tube feeding syndrome in head and neck surgery. *Archives of Otolaryngology,* 1969, *89,* 533–536.

Welsh, J. D. Isolated lactase deficiency in humans: Report on 100 patients. *Medicine,* 1970, *49,* 257–277.

**Primary research articles that should be reviewed to understand adequately the research base for this protocol. These articles may be found in Chapter 3. It is suggested that these articles be read in the following order: (1) Walike et al., 1975; (2) Walike and Walike, 1973; and (3) Walike and Walike, 1977.*

Supplement A: Selected Annotated Bibliography[5]

Bayless, T. M., & Rosensweig, N. S. A racial difference in incidence of lactase deficiency. *Journal of the American Medical Association,* 1966, *197,* 138–142.

(Author abstract.) An incidence survey of milk intolerance and lactase deficiency was conducted in 40 healthy nonpatient volunteers. There were 20 blacks and 20 whites. Nineteen of the 20 black subjects and two of the 20 white subjects gave a history of milk intolerance. The majority had noted the onset during or after adolescence. Lactose intolerance occurred in 20 of the 21 milk-intolerant subjects; 18 of the 20 were black. There was also a prominent racial difference in the incidence of low levels of intestinal lactase activity. Deficient levels were observed in 70 percent of the 20 blacks, in contrast to only one of the 20 whites. These data strongly favor a genetic etiology for the isolated lactase deficiencies seen so commonly in adults.

Bayless, T. M., Rothfeld, B., Massa, C., Wise, L., Paige, D., & Bedine, M. S. Lactose and milk intolerance: Clinical implications. *The New England Journal of Medicine,* 1975, *292,* 1156–1159.

(Author abstract.) We studied 166 hospitalized male patients to determine the clinical importance of tolerance-test–determined "lactose intolerance," assumed to affect most of the world's adults. Abnormal lactose tolerance tests were found in 81 percent of 98 blacks, 12 percent of 59 whites of Scandinavian or Northwestern European extraction, and 3 of 9 non-European whites. Seventy-two percent of the "lactose-intolerant" subjects had previously realized that milk drinking could induce abdominal and bowel symptoms. Two hundred forty milliliters of low-fat milk produced gaseousness or cramps in 59 percent of 44 "lactose-intolerant" men, and 68 percent were symptomatic with the equivalent amount of lactose. None of 18 "lactose-tolerant" men noted symptoms with milk or lactose. Refusal to drink 240 ml of low-fat milk

[5]*These articles were not reviewed in the protocol and are not reprinted in Chapter 3. They were selected for annotation because they may hold special interest for some readers.*

served with meals correlated significantly with "lactose-intolerance": 31.4 percent versus 12.9 percent among "lactose-tolerant" patients.

"Lactose intolerance" is common in adults and is a clinically relevant problem.

Bedine, M. S., & Bayless, M.D. Intolerance of small amounts of lactose by individuals with low lactase levels. *Gastroenterology,* 1973, *65,* 735–743.

This research was conducted in two parts: (1) "To study more clinically relevant amounts of lactose and the apparent variation in milk and lactose intolerance, adults with low intestinal lactase levels and milk intolerance were fed varying amounts of lactose to determine their threshold for symptoms" (p. 736); (2) "To determine if measurable derangements in fluid and electrolyte absorption occur with small doses of lactose, changes in net fluid movement and electrolyte concentrations in the small intestine, after feeding 3 to 24 g of lactose, were determined by intraluminal intubation studies" (p. 736). Among 20 subjects with low lactase levels, 75 percent were found to have symptoms of flatulence, distention, cramps, loose bowel movements, or diarrhea with 12 g of lactose (equivalent to 8 ounces of milk) or less. The authors also present "objective evidence of fluid and sodium accumulation in the small bowel with these small lactose loads" (p. 735).

Gault, M. H., Dixon, M. E., Doyle, M., & Cohen, W. M. Hypernatremia, azotemia, and dehydration due to high-protein tube feeding. *Annals of Internal Medicine,* 1968, *68,* 778–791.

(Journal summary.) Severe dehydration, hypernatremia and hyponatruria, and azotemia in marked excess of creatinemia developed in three patients given high-protein tube feedings. The patients were fully conscious when tube feeding was instituted, and each had a tracheostomy coincidental to treatment of carcinoma of the larynx or oral cavity.

In two cases, several features demonstrated that the hypernatremia was due predominantly to dehydration and not to excess salt.

In patients who are unconscious or who for other reasons are unable to experience, communicate, or alleviate their thirst, this syndrome may develop rapidly when fluid losses are increased, and tube-feeding water protein ratios may be higher than those ordinarily well tolerated. A similar degree of care should be exercised in the regulation of constituents and the monitoring of fluid and electrolyte balance with the use of tube feedings as is done when intravenous therapy is given.

Hanson, R. L., Walike, B. C., Grant, M., Kubo, W., Bergstrom, N., Padilla, G., & Wong, H. L. Patient responses and problems associated with tube feeding. *Washington State Journal of Nursing,* Winter 1975, 9–13.

The purpose of this study was to assess current practices in tube feeding, to determine the nature and prevalence of the problems associated with tube feeding, and to gain insight into the areas in which further research is needed. The sample consisted of 121 patients receiving tube feedings for a total of 1730 days. Most of the data was collected retrospectively from patient charts. Data concerning gastrointestinal responses to tube feeding and patient weight, as well as fluid and electrolyte balance, are discussed.

This article is an abridged version of the study findings presented by Walike, et al. in *Communicating Nursing Research,* 1975.

Johnson, J. D., Kretchmer, N., & Simoons, F. J. Lactose malabsorption: Its biology and history. *Advances in Pediatrics,* 1974, *21,* 197–237.

This paper discusses the biochemical, physiologic, geographic, and social aspects of lactose malabsorption. It provides an extensive review of the literature in a very readable style. Recommended for those with a special interest in this topic.

Jones, E. S., & Peaston, M.J.T. Metabolic care during acute illnesses. *The Practitioner,* 1966, *196,* 271–275.

(Author summary.) Experiences in three departments of a district hospital indicated the need for improved metabolic care of adult patients during acute illnesses. Techniques are described which have enabled the authors to provide adequate nutrition and metabolic balance for a large number of patients. The foods used were milk powder, fat emulsion, amino acids, and sugars, given intragastrically or intravenously.

Kubo, W., Grant, M., Walike, B., Bergstrom, N., Wong, H., Hanson, R., & Padilla, G. Fluid and electrolyte problems of tube-fed patients. *American Journal of Nursing,* 1976, *76,* 912–916.

Discussion of the fluid and electrolyte problems found by an assessment of tube-fed patients. Data collection in this study covered a total of 1730 tube-feeding days for 121 patients. Laboratory statistics are presented for the total sample. Within-patient analysis

(analysis of individual patient problems) is presented for two cases. Implications for nursing practice are discussed.

Minckley, B. B. Critique of "patient problems related to tube feeding." In M. V. Batey (Ed.), *Communicating Nursing Research* (vol. 7). Boulder, Colo.: WICHE, 1975.

Critique of the Walike et al. (1975) study on patient problems related to tube feeding. The Walike et al. study appears in the same volume.

Pareira, M. D. *Therapeutic nutrition with tube feeding.* Springfield, Ill.: Chas C Thomas, 1959.

This study is no longer current, but it remains interesting for the incidence rate of diarrhea which is reported. Of 316 patients receiving a milk-based mixture as their sole intake (240 by tube and 76 orally), diarrhea is reported to have developed in 22 (7 percent).

Rosenberg, F. H. Lactose intolerance. *American Journal of Nursing,* 1977, *77,* 823–824.

A brief and concise review of some of the literature on lactose intolerance is presented. The prevalence and population distribution of lactose tolerance are discussed; symptomatology is reviewed; diagnostic tests are cited; and implications for therapeutic diet changes are made.

Walike, B. C. Disturbances of food intake and nutrition. In H. Moidel, B. Wagner, & E. Giblin (Eds.), *Nursing care of the patient with medical–surgical disorders* (2nd ed.). New York: McGraw-Hill Co., 1976.

The discussion on tube feeding and tube-feeding diets is relevant to protocol users.

Walike, B. C., Walike, J. W., Hanson, R. L., Grant, M., Kubo, W., Bergstrom, N., Wong, H. L., Padilla, G., & Williams, K. Nasogastric tube feeding: Clinical complications and current progress of research. *Northwest Health Team Approach,* 1975, *2*(6), 33–41.

(Authors' abstract.) The present series of studies has indicated problems of patient welfare and comfort associated with nasogastric tube feedings, including inadequate caloric intake, nasal and oropharyngeal discomfort, diarrhea, constipation, nausea, borborygmi, anxiety, and dehydration. The causes of some of these problems have been identified; others remain to be studied. A relative intolerance for the large amount of lactose (milk sugar) frequently contained in tube-feeding diets contributes to diarrhea. The temperature of the diet at administration has no effect either on its tolerance or on the occurrence of diarrhea, and only slight effect on patient comfort. Inadequate hydration in association with compromised renal function, especially in elderly patients, can accelerate dehydration. Current concepts of optimal nasogastric tube feeding management are presented, and the causes and possible methods for alleviation of several specific disturbances from nasogastric tube feedings are described.

Walike, J. W. Tube-feeding syndrome in head and neck surgery. *Archives of Otolaryngology,* 1969, *89,* 533–536.

(Author summary.) The tube-feeding syndrome consists of dehydration, hypernatremia, hyperchloremia, and azotemia. It is a complication of feeding a patient excessively high solute loads or not providing sufficient additional water to utilize usual tube-feeding diets. This complication is most apt to occur in elderly patients who have compromised renal function. A case of this syndrome is presented, which occurred in a head and neck patient. The increased use of tube-feeding diets in head and neck patients prompted this report. The clinical features, laboratory data, physiology, treatment, and prevention of this syndrome are presented.

Welsh, J. D. Isolated lactase deficiency in humans: Report on 100 patients. *Medicine,* 1970, *49,* 257–277.

Analysis of data on 100 subjects with an isolated lactase deficiency and 150 with normal lactase activity is done in order "to establish criteria for the diagnosis of a lactose malabsorption and as a basis for substantiation of the importance of this clinical entity as a cause of symptoms."

Supplement B: Stool-Consistency Diagrams*

1. watery

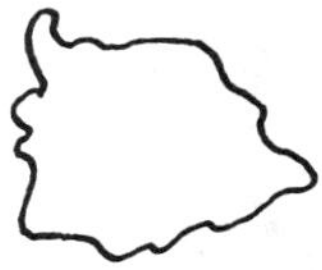

2. liquid, creamy

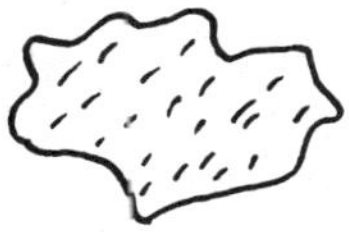

3. very loose, mushy, semiliquid

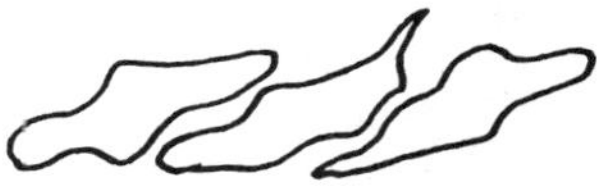

4. loose, soft

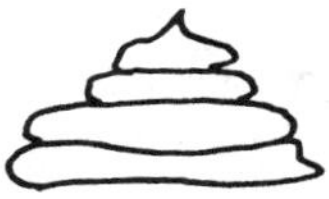

5. formed w/some liquid

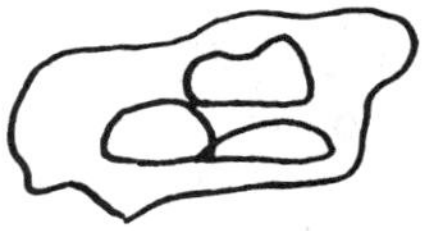

6. soft, formed

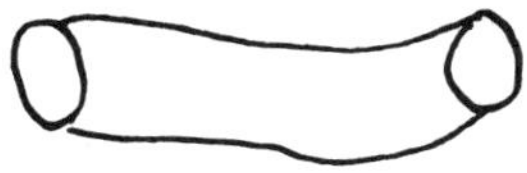

7. normal, formed

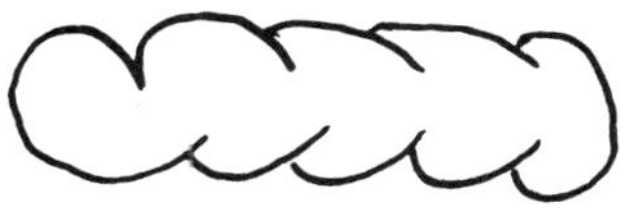

8. hard

9. hard, dry

*Used with permission of B. Walike Hansen, Tube-feeding Project, University of Michigan, 1978.

Supplement C: Suggested Evaluation Procedure

Evaluation is an essential component of any innovation which is implemented in the practice setting. To yield meaningful results, the evaluation should be carefully planned and systematically conducted. The variables which need to be measured in order to evaluate the lactose-free diet have been specified in the protocol. The methods and tools presented in this supplement are intended to guide staff in the evaluation process.

Patient Data Collection Card

A patient data-collection form or card should be kept on each patient in the baseline and postimplementation groups. Figure 1 shows an example of such a card. The card guides the collection of data on variables which may influence or help explain the results of the trial. Some of these variables can be used to compare the baseline and postimplementation groups to ensure a reasonable degree of similarity between them; examples of these variables include race and diagnosis. Variables such as age and type of tube can be used to ensure comparability to the research-base population. Other variables may be used to interpret individual data. Stool history, for example, provides an individual baseline which can be used to ascertain whether a client returned to his or her "normal" while on the lactose-free diet. A client's usual stool consistency can be determined by interview and assigned an approximate rating.

It should be noted that, in certain cases, clients may stay on tube feedings for the duration of a lengthy hospital admission, or even indefinitely. It is possible for these long-term patients to be on lactose-containing diets during the baseline period and then be placed on lactose-free diets in the implementation period. Data may be collected on the same patient in both periods, and this is not problematic for the evaluation. To avoid confusion, however, these patients will need two data-collection cards (that is, one for each evaluation period).

ADDRESSOGRAPH

TUBE FEEDING

PATIENT DATA CARD

Trial Phase __________

AGE _____ RACE or ETHNICITY __________

DIAGNOSIS: (1) __________

(2) __________

TYPE OF TUBE __________ ON TUBE FEEDINGS SINCE __________ (Date)

STOOL HX: Average No. of Stools/Day __________

Usual Consistency (Rating) __________

DATES ON DATA COLLECTION: Start _____ Finish _____

PROCESS COMMENTS: __________

Fig. 1. Patient data-collection card.

Bedside Tube-Feeding Data-Collection Form

The bedside tube-feeding data-collection form (Table 1) can be used to collect information on the dependent variables in both the baseline and postimplementation periods. The stool-consistency rating scale listed on the form needs to be used in conjunction with the stool-consistency diagrams (see Supplement B). A decision about how to collect data on gastrointestinal complaints will need to be made in order to use the form efficiently. In addition to indicating patient complaints about symptoms only when they are offered, it may be efficient to ask patients once each day whether they have experienced these symptoms (nausea, burping, and so forth) in the past 24 hours.

Data should be collected for 5 to 7 days on each patient in each evaluation period. A new data-collection form should be used for each 24-hour period. When a patient has been on the assigned

Table 1
Bedside Tube-Feeding Data-Collection Form[1]

ADDRESSOGRAPH

Pt. Study Day ____________
Date ____/____/____
Trial Phase ____________

INSTRUCTIONS: Begin a new section below with each scheduled tube feeding. All other entries should be made in the spaces to the right of the most recent feeding. Intake, Urine Output, and Emesis should be recorded in terms of volume for each occurrence. Each occurrence of a stool should be indicated by a check (√) in the "Occur" column and indication of the consistency by entry of the corresponding number from the scale shown below:

1 = Watery
2 = Liquid, creamy
3 = Very loose, mushy, semiliquid
4 = Loose, soft
5 = Formed with some liquid
6 = Soft, formed
7 = Normal, formed
8 = Hard
9 = Hard, dry

The occurrence of all other items should be indicated by a check (√) in the respective column.

TUBE FEEDINGS		OTHER INTAKE (Specify kind and incl. H_2O to irrig. tube)	URINE OUTPUT (cc)	EMESIS (cc)	STOOL		COMPLAINTS OF OR OBSERVED								
TIME	VOLUME (cc)	CC TYPE			Occurrence	Consistency	Nausea	Burping	Gurgling Bowel Sound	Pass Flatus	Distention "Gas"	Fullness	Heartburn	Cramps	Vol (cc) Refused

Please record any comments on the back of this form.

[1] Adapted and used with permission of B. Walike Hansen, Tube-feeding Project, University of Michigan, 1978.

Table 2
Summarized Tube-Feeding Data

Trial Phase: ______
Diet: ______
Dates: ______

NAME AND/OR ID	AGE	RACE OR ETHNICITY	DIAGNOSIS	STOOL HISTORY		% DAYS ON MEDICATIONS						TUBE FEEDINGS		EMESIS	STOOL		% DAYS COMPLAINED OF								
				Av. No. Per Day	*Usual Consistency Rating*	*Antacids*	*Antibiotics*	*Iron*	*Laxatives*	*Antidiarrhetics*	*Other*	*Av. Per Day*	*Av. Vol Per Day*	*Av. Vol Per Day*	*Av. No. Per Day*	*Usual Consistency Rating*	*Nausea*	*Burping*	*Gurgling*	*Flatulence*	*Distention—"Gas"*	*Fullness*	*Heartburn*	*Cramps*	*Av. Vol Tube Feeding Refused Per Day*
1.																									
2.																									
3.																									
4.																									
5.																									
6.																									
7.																									
8.																									
9.																									
10.																									
Totals and averages:																									

Note: Percentage of days $= \frac{\text{No. of days with (X) occurring}}{\text{Total no. of days observed in trial phase}} \times 100.$

For example, percentage of days on antacids $= \frac{\text{No. of days on antacids}}{\text{No. of days observed in trial phase}} \times 100.$

diet for 7 days and/or when the patient is discharged, information on the bedside data sheets and patient data card should be summarized.

Summary Form

A form for summarizing the data in each trial period has been designed, and some may find it useful in doing the basic calculations. Use of such a form has the advantage of summarizing the data on a few sheets of paper, as well as making a visual display of the data for colleagues (see Table 2).

Comparison of the baseline and postimplementation data summaries will yield information about the similarity of the groups on age, ethnicity, diagnosis, stool history, and recent medication pattern. Stool history and medication pattern may also be used to explain unexpected results. For instance, if the incidence of diarrhea in patients receiving the lactose-containing diet seems low, it might be attributable to a large amount of antidiarrhetic medications.

Comparison of the baseline and postimplementation data summaries will show the effect of the innovation on the primary dependent variables of stool frequency and stool consistency, as well as on the optional variables (other gastrointestinal symptoms). From such comparisons, it should be possible to determine the benefit of the innovation in the clinical setting.

Chapter 3
RESEARCH BASE

PATIENT PROBLEMS RELATED TO TUBE FEEDING*

Barbara C. Walike, Ph.D., Geraldine Padilla, Ph.D., Nancy Bergstrom, M.S., Robert L. Hanson, M.N., Winifred Kubo, M.S.N., Marcia Grant, M.S.N., and Hilda Luna Wong, M.A.

Nasogastric tube feedings were first recorded as an alternative to oral alimentation in 1598.[32] Their use is increasing due to a growing recognition of the role of inadequate nutrition in delayed healing and recovery, more frequent radical surgery, and improved methods for maintaining other vital functions. The administration of tube feedings has been associated with frequent problems for both the patient and the nurse. Although life-threatening disturbances, such as significant shifts in fluid and electrolyte balance and aspira-

*Barbara C. Walike, Ph.D.: Assistant Professor, Schools of Nursing and Medicine, University of Washington; Geraldine Padilla, Ph.D.: Director of Nursing Research, City of Hope National Medical Center; Nancy Bergstrom, M.S.: Assistant Professor, School of Nursing, University of San Francisco, Robert L. Hanson, M.N.: Director,

tion of liquid diet, are relatively rare, numerous problems of patient discomfort and gastrointestinal distress have been described.

The purpose of this study was to assess the nature of problems associated with tube feedings and to obtain an indication of their prevalence. The ultimate aim was to develop testable hypotheses concerning potential methods of reducing or eliminating the identified and potential problems.

OVERVIEW OF THE STUDY

A comprehensive literature review focused upon the reported indications of tube feedings, the demographic characteristics of tube-fed patients, the rationale and recommendations concerning method of administration, the contents and handling of the tube-feeding diets, and the complications and patient responses to tube feedings. Inadequacies of information on all of these topics led to the design and execution of a large-scale survey of patients receiving tube feedings in order to provide better information concerning both current practices and problem areas.

A study of 121 patients receiving tube feedings for a total of 1730 days was conducted by 7 investigators in 3 western states—California, Hawaii, and Washington. A total of 145 variables were identified, and data on these were collected daily or at specified intervals for up to 20 days per patient. The primary source of data was the patient chart, with supplemental information derived from

---

Nursing Research, Virginia Mason Hospital and Clinical Assistant Professor, School of Nursing, University of Washington; Winifred Kubo, M.S.N.: Assistant Professor, School of Nursing, University of Hawaii; Marcia Grant, M.S.N.: Assistant Professor, School of Nursing, University of Hawaii; and Hilda Luna Wong, M.A.: Associate Professor, School of Nursing, Loma Linda University.

This study was supported by NIH Grants NU00415, Regional Program for Nursing Research and Development; AM16217, Obesity and the Regulation of Appetite; NU00369, Action Program in Nursing Research Facilitation; and Ross Laboratories and the Northwest Medical Research Foundation, Inc.

We are grateful to all of those who assisted us in data collection and computer analysis, including Lynne Kalnasy, Verlene Vanderberg, the research staff at the City of Hope National Medical Center, and the staff of the WICHE office.

Reprinted with permission from Batey, M. V. (ed.): Communicating nursing research: Critical issues in access to data. *Boulder, Colorado: Western Interstate Commission for Higher Education, 1975. Presented at Communicating Nursing Research Conference.*

the nursing staff and from 41 patients who were in the hospital during data collection.

Data were collected in a variety of clinical settings, including private hospitals, large university medical centers, public hospitals, extended care facilities, and nursing homes located in large and small cities. Patients included all major racial groups and many categories of diagnoses.

Computer analysis of these data, supplemented by additional case studies, has led to a description of current tube-feeding regimens of associated, although not necessarily causally related, problems and of areas requiring systematic investigation in order to effect improved patient care.

Because of the broad scope of this study, which involves physical, physiological, and psychological assessments, this discussion will be presented in a somewhat unorthodox manner. The method of data collection, including the development of tools and selection of patients, will be presented first. The remainder of the paper will review the three major areas covered by both the literature reviews and findings of the present study: (1) characteristics of patients receiving tube feedings, (2) procedures used in the administration of tube feedings, and (3) patient responses to tube feedings. Under each of these topics the findings of previous studies, together with the results of this study, will be presented and discussed.

METHOD OF DATA COLLECTION AND ANAYLSIS

Although much of the literature concerning the methods and types of tube feeding indicated that problems could occur, no documentation of either the incidence or causes of these problems was found. In the process of a systematic review of the literature, each of the investigators developed a list of variables that were suggested to directly or interactively determine the success of tube feeding. An earlier set of forms developed for an experimental study of tube feedings was greatly modified and expanded to include all variables that might be relevant.[41] Because of the survey nature of this study, no attempt was made to reduce or limit the number of variables. For two reasons, all variables were included whether or not the data were likely to be readily available on any particular item. First, even a small amount of data on a particular question (for example, length of tube insertion) could be useful in planning for future studies; and second, it was hoped that the same forms, together with the computer programs developed for their analysis, could be used beyond this initial survey in experimental studies that might be indicated from the present results.

The 145 variables identified for inclusion in the study were sorted into five types of forms according to how often each variable was to be assessed. The five groups of data were as follows:

1. *Study period constants.* Largely demographic data, including physical and health status; collected once for each subject.
2. *Variables recorded daily.* Detailed data concerning the patient's tube-feeding method, diet, intake and output, and vital signs.
3. *Variables recorded periodically.* Data collected on days 1, 3, 5, 9, 14, and 19, and reflective of each interval; they included physical and emotional status, drug therapy, and attitude toward and reaction to the diet.
4. *Chemistry data..* All available blood chemistry data during the tube-feeding period, plus one report prior to tube feeding if available.
5. *Hematology and urine data.* All available hematology, blood gas, and urine chemistry data during the tube feeding, plus one report prior to tube feeding if available.

The following definitions of terms are used in this report. *Patient* refers to the 121 individuals in the sample. *Study days* refers to the 1730 total days of tube feeding. *Periodic days* refers to data collected on days 1, 3, 5, 9, 14, and 19. The maximum number of periodic days reported is 744.

A pilot study of three to six patients was conducted by each investigator prior to finalizing the data-collection forms. The investigators modified and clarified the tools and developed standardized, triplicate data-collection forms, which were formated and coded for keypunching. Explicit guidelines for the data-collection procedure were developed to insure the greatest consistency in method. Periodic meetings of the investigators were held to review the procedures and to resolve any difficulties arising during data collection and analysis.

Data collection for each patient was initiated with one recording of baseline blood chemistry, hematology, and urine chemistry determination prior to the onset of tube feeding when these were available. Data were collected from the onset of tube feeding through the last day of tube feeding, or to the twentieth day, whichever occurred first.

One copy of all data was forwarded to a central location where all keypunching and computer analysis were performed. An initial printout of all data was checked for accuracy by each investigator. A FORTRAN program was written to collate all data, and subsequent analysis used the Statistical Package for the Social Sciences. Additional analysis of diet contents and other uncoded data was carried out manually by each investigator.

PATIENT SAMPLE CHARACTERISTICS

Demographic Data

Demographic data on tube-fed patients are virtually nonexistent. The kinds of statistical information released by such agencies as the National Center for Health Statistics are inadequate to determine the characteristics of tube-fed patients. Conspicuously missing from the health-disease literature or the literature on tube feeding is any description by race, culture, age, sex, eating habits, bowel habits, or even diagnoses of tube-fed patients. Thus, there are no data to which the present patient sample characteristics could be compared.

Included in this project were 121 patients receiving tube feedings for a total of 1730 days at 4 major medical centers and 21 smaller hospitals and extended care facilities. There were 48 females and 73 males in the sample (Table 1), of which 69 percent were Caucasian, 19 percent Oriental, 7 percent brown (primarily Polynesian), and 4 percent Black. Patients ranged in age from 14 to 90 years.

Physical Status and Diagnoses

Although primary diagnoses were varied (Table 2), head and neck carcinoma (40 percent) and central nervous system deficits (32 percent) were predominant. Of the sample, 81 percent had had surgery, and of these, 39 percent had head and neck surgery. Prior to the study, 36 percent of the patients had received radiation ther-

Table 1
Summary of Demographic Characteristics of 121 Patients

CHARACTERISTIC	NO.	%
Sex		
Females	48	40
Males	73	60
Age		
14–25	5	4
26–35	4	3
36–45	9	7
46–55	16	13
56–65	40	33
66–75	21	18
76–85	19	16
86–95	7	6
Race		
Caucasian	84	69
Oriental	23	19
Brown	9	7
Black	5	4

apy. The physical condition of the patients during the study period was classified as "fair" or "poor" for 72 percent; 25 percent of the patients were considered to be in "good" condition.

Periodic data collected during the study revealed that patients were alert and conscious on 51 percent of the study days (Table 3), were conscious but confused or were semiconscious on 32 percent of the study days, and were comatose on 16 percent of the study days. On 48 percent of the study days, patients were able to be ambulatory, at least briefly. The emotional or psychological sta-

Table 2
Summary of Physical Status and Diagnosis

DATA TYPE	PATIENTS FROM WHOM DATA OBTAINED (NO.)	STATUS	NO.	%
Primary diagnosis	121	Head and neck carcinoma	48	40
		Nervous system deficits	39	32
		Other	34	28
Surgery	98	Head and neck surgery	38	39
		Other	60	61
Physical condition during study period	121	Fair or poor	87	72
		Good	30	25
		Excellent	4	3

Table 3
Summary of Patient Consciousness, Pain, and Nervousness Levels

DATA TYPE	PERIODIC DAYS OBSERVATIONS (RECORDED NO.)	STATUS	NO.	%
Consciousness state	744	Alert and conscious	380	51
		Conscious and confused, semiconscious	238	32
		Comatose	119	16
		Other	7	1
Emotional state	389	Calm	187	48
		Some nervousness	152	39
		Extreme nervousness	47	12
		Other	3	1
Pain	744	Mild to moderate	164	22
		Severe	29	4
		Pain severity not noted	149	20
		Other	402	54

tus of the patients was recorded on 389 of the 744 periodic data-collection days. On 48 percent of those days, patients were reported to be calm, some degree of nervousness was reported on 39 percent of the days, and extreme nervousness was reported on 12 percent of the days. Pain was described as mild to moderate on 22 percent of the days and severe on 4 percent. Pain was present but its severity was not specified on an additional 20 percent of the days. Thus, the typical patient in this tube-fed sample was on bed-rest in fair or poor condition and was experiencing some pain and nervousness. All of these characteristics interact closely with the success and outcomes of tube feedings.

Medical History

Information relating to the patient's medical and surgical history and personal habits that might have influenced subject response to tube feedings were reported as often as they appeared in the patient record or were available from direct contact with the patient. Of the patients, 43 percent were known to have had surgery prior to this hospitalization. Ten patients had a history of hemorrhoids; 7 of these reported prior hemorrhoid surgery. Reported gastrointestinal disorders included a history of gastrectomy (3 patients), gall bladder disorders (4), and ulcers (14). Fifteen patients reported having diabetes and 2 patients reported some previous thyroid disorder. A history of renal disease was noted for 9 subjects.

Data regarding weight changes were available for 72 patients. Fifty-eight percent (N = 42) reported a weight loss of more than 10 pounds in the 6 months prior to tube feeding, 39 percent (N = 28) reported no significant weight change, and 3 percent (N = 2) reported a weight gain of more than 10 pounds in the preceding 6-month period.

The bowel habits of the patients were known for 57 of the 121 in the sample. Of the 57 patients, 42 percent (24) indicated regular bowel habits, 47 percent (27) indicated they were sometimes or often constipated, and 9 percent (5) indicated they had frequent diarrhea.

The use of laxatives was reported by 34 percent of the sample, and more than half of those used them one to two times a week. Four patients reported the use of enemas from once a day to two times a month.

Data regarding the history of smoking were recorded for 73 of the 121 subjects. Fifteen of the 73 patients had never smoked; however, the remaining 58 were former smokers (26) or were currently smoking moderately to heavily (30).

In summary, tube-fed patients in this study were men and women of all races; the largest group was Caucasian men. The primary reasons for tube feeding included head and neck carcinoma and central nervous system deficits. Most had a recent history of weight loss and were limited in their activity level.

Interacting Effects of Medications

In any evaluation of responses to tube feeding, the interaction of concurrent medications with many of the subject variables must be considered. The interactive effects of tube feeding and medications are greatest in two areas: (1) consciousness state, level of confusion, and sedation, and (2) gastrointestinal responses, particularly with reference to stool frequency. Antibiotics have been associated with both diarrhea and constipation. Analgesics of some types have been associated with constipation in non-tube-fed subjects. Thus, data concerning both the frequency and amount of medication administration must be considered an important variable in studying the complications of tube-feeding patients.

The frequency with which each category of drugs was administered during the study period for each patient is shown in Table

Table 4
Use of Drugs During Study Period

DRUG CATEGORY	PERCENTAGE OF STUDY PERIOD DAYS DRUG GIVEN TO PATIENTS*
Antibiotic	68
Analgesic	38
Laxative or suppository	27
Antacid	22
Tranquilizer	16
Sedative	14
Diuretic	9
Antidiarrhea	7

* Derived from 744 periodic data days.

4. Patients receiving antibiotics experienced the same range of stool consistency as those without antibiotics. The distribution of stool consistency is so similar that it does not seem to be affected appreciably by antibiotics as a group, although individual antibiotics may have had some effects. Specific interactive effects have not yet been analyzed.

TUBE-FEEDING PROCEDURES AND DIETS

The procedure of tube feeding involves a great many factors that both singly and in combination affect the success of tube feeding. These include type of tube, method of administration, frequency and volumes of feedings, and contents of diets. Consideration will be given to each of these aspects of tube feeding, with the recognition that these factors interact.

Tube Characteristics

Tubes suggested for use with nasogastric tube feedings vary primarily in four respects: length, material, location and number of eyes, and lumen size. Sizes recommended range from "thin" [46,10] to a number 16 French.[5] Rubber,[40] plastic,[36] polyvinyl, and polyethylene[2] are the most frequent materials mentioned. A preference for polyethylene was stated by Barron because it stays soft and flexible in contrast to polyvinyl,[2] which tends to become hard and can be irritating, and by Wohl,[46] who noted that a thin polyethylene

Table 5
Summary of Common Characteristics of Commercially Available Nasogastric Feeding Tubes*

CHARACTERISTIC	DETAIL
French sizes	5, 6, 8, 10, 12, 14, 16, 18
Lengths (in.)	15, 30, 36, 42, 48, 50
Number of eyes	2, 4 (usually spaced 1 in. apart)
Tube material	Clear plastic, red rubber
Connectors	
Material	Rubber, plastic, latex
Types	Flared, Luer
Graduated markings (in.)	18, 22, 26, 30; or 10, 20, 30

* Nearly any combination of above detail characteristics is available.

tube is well tolerated and may be left in place for as long as 4 months without problems of clogging or irritation.

Other tubes recommended for tube feeding have unique characteristics, such as a mercury-filled rubber balloon attached to the end of the tube to facilitate its passage.[10] Taylor suggested the use of a number 16 French rubber urethral catheter (we question use of such a catheter, normally 12 to 14 inches long, because of the probable esophageal location of the tube tip).[40] Table 5 contains descriptive data on commercially available feeding tubes. As is apparent, they differ in diameter, length, number of lumen, material and even markings. Table 6 indicates the distribution of the various types of tubes found in this study. The sizes of tubes are indicated in Table 7. Of the patients with known nasogastric tube sizes 70 percent had number 12 to number 16 French tubes.

Patient Position during Feeding

Sutton recommended that the patient should be in a sitting or a semi-Fowlers position for the nasogastric feeding, and a flat po-

Table 6
Type of Nasogastric Tubes

MATERIAL	PATIENTS (NO.)
"Plastic"	42
"Rubber"	25
Polyvinyl	5
Unknown	49

Table 7
Size of Feeding Tubes

FRENCH SIZE	NO.	%
6	1	2
8	1	2
10	3	5
12	5	8
14	9	15
16	33	56
18	6	10
20	1	2
Greater than 20 or unknown	23	

sition for a gastrostomy feeding.[39] Noyes, Camp, and van Sickel mentioned sitting in a chair as a possible position for nasogastric feeding but noted a preference for a supine position.[30] Very little is known about the relative advisability of various positions during tube feedings. In this study, the positions of patients during tube feedings were recorded on 332 of the 1730 feeding days. During this time, the head of the bed was elevated 30° on 36 percent of the days and the beds were elevated 45° on 54 percent of the days. The supine or sitting position was noted occasionally.

Gastric Aspiration

There is no agreement among other authors as to the advisability of gastric aspiration prior to tube feeding, and the disposition of the aspirant—that is, its reinjection or disposal. Some have recommended reducing the following tube feeding by the amount aspirated, while others suggest using gastric aspiration only to ascertain the location of the tube tip. In this study, gastric aspiration was known to have been performed on 52 days; however, data did not reveal the fate of the gastric aspirant. It was known, however, that at least for a few patients, the gastric aspirant was discarded prior to infusing the next feeding.

Rate of Administration

Authors who mentioned rate usually did so with precaution against too rapid administration[37,18,6,29] to prevent distention and nausea.[18] A factor affecting the rate of administration is whether

Table 8
Rate of Administration of Tube Feedings*

DURATION OF INFUSION (MIN.)	STUDY DAYS (%)
Less than 5	61
5–15	30
15–30	5
Over 30	3

* N = 778 patient days.

the feeding is administered by gravity or by force. The authors who recommended a slow rate generally advocated the gravity or continuous pump method. Kozier and DuGas and Saunders et al., none of whom specifically advocated a slow rate, indicated that slight pressure using a syringe might be necessary and acceptable.[24,36] Brunner et al., however, stated that force should never be used, but gave no explanation.[6] Hanson, in a study of tube feeding using normal subjects, found an increased incidence of accelerated heart rate, nausea, gagging, and regurgitation associated with forced or rapid feedings.[19]

Data concerning the duration of tube feedings were available on 778 of 1730 study period days. On 61 percent of these study days, tube feedings were administered in less than 5 minutes. Table 8 contains the rate of administration of the remaining tube feedings. No patients were on continuous feeding. As illustrated in Table 9, the percentage of patients receiving tube feedings in 5 minutes or less increased as the number of days of tube feeding increased.

Table 9
Duration of Tube Feedings*

	PERCENTAGES OF DURATION OF FEEDING TIMES		
DAY	*0–5 Min.*	*5–15 Min.*	*15–30 Min.*
1	58.2	27.3	5.5
5	56	34	8
10	58	34	5
15	74	22	4
20	70	25	5

* N = 778 patient days.

Temperature of Administration

Many "house" formula tube feedings are prepared in advance and refrigerated prior to their administration. Whether the refrigerated feedings should be warmed prior to administration is not agreed upon in the literature. Several authors indicated that the feeding should be warmed to room or body temperature or higher.[43,40,39,35,24,12,6,38,29] Only three of these works provided explanations. Kozier and DuGas stated that "food that is at body temperature is most easily tolerated."[24] White, Rubino, and De Lorey and Fuerst and Wolff indicated that warming the feeding is necessary to prevent the patient from chilling.[43,12] Horsch questioned the clinical justification for warming the feeding,[21] and Fason[11] and Phipps and Barker[34] stated they observed no adverse effects from administering a cold feeding. Holt et al. found no adverse effects from feeding cold formula to premature infants,[20] and Hanson found no relationship between the temperature of a tube feeding and the response of normal adult subjects.[19] Hanson also demonstrated that when a 250-cc feeding, begun at refrigerated temperature, is given over a period of 30 minutes, the feeding is near body temperature by the time it reaches the stomach. Williams and Walike demonstrated only minimal effects of cold tube feeding on gastric motility and gastric emptying in primates.[44]

Observations concerning the temperature of tube feedings were recorded on 869 of the 1730 study period days. Feedings were administered at room temperature on 83 percent of the days, were warmed to body temperature on 14 percent of the days, and were administered cold on 3 percent of the days. Patients who received tube feedings for the longest number of days were most likely to receive the feedings at room temperature. Very few feedings were warmed on the twentieth day of tube feeding.

Number of Feedings per Day

Varied frequencies of tube feeding are recommended in the literature, ranging from continuous feedings[3] to several times per day. The most frequent recommendation is in the range of every 3 to 4 hours.[24,35,39,40,43] Frequent and small or continuous feedings are recommended by some authors, usually with the rationale of preventing nausea, abdominal distention, diarrhea, or other gastrointestinal disturbances.[36,46,24,37,3]

In this study, by far the greatest amount of data relating to the procedure of tube feeding concerned the number of feedings administered per day (known for 1563 of 1730 days). Only one to three feedings per study day were reported 13 percent (N = 198) of the time, and as many as seven or more feedings per study day were reported on 13 percent (N = 199) of the days. Patients received four to six feedings per day on 63 percent (N = 915) of the feeding days. (No feedings or more than 10 feedings account for the remaining 11 percent of the patient days.) Most feedings were given by gravity from a reservoir whose height was 20 to 25 inches.

Volume of Diet Intake

The volume of a feeding is dependent on the frequency and number of feedings and the total intake; however, the typical recommended volume is 150 to 300 cc.[43,40,39,35,37] Sutton[39] and White, Rubino, and De Lorey[43] warned that the volume of a single feeding should not exceed 500 cc. Nursing journals and texts generally recommend that tube feedings should be given at frequent intervals and in small quantities. Nursing practice, as reflected in this study, followed those recommendations closely. Data for the

Table 10
Comparison Between Number of Feedings per Day and Mean Volume of Diet Intake for 24 Hr.

FEEDINGS (NO.)	MEAN INTAKE (24 HR.)	MEAN INTAKE PER FEEDING	STUDY DAYS* (%)
2	641	320	4
3	977	325	7
4	1142	285	21
5	1463	292	18
6	1574	262	24
7	1784	254	5
8	1634	204	6
9	1481	164	1
10	2028	202	1
11	1555	141	.7
12	1569	130	4
13	3220	247	.07
14	2000	142	.07
24	521	21	.7

* N = 1,394 study days.

first day of tube feeding are not included in the following discussion because the first day tended to be highly variable.

The highest mean volume per feeding was 325 cc given three times per day to 11 subjects. In Table 10 a comparison is made of the number of feedings per day to the mean volume of intake for 24 hours. The patients receiving 24 feedings per day reflected the presence of an "ulcer regimen."

It was found that the number of feedings and the total volume tended to increase up to seven to eight feedings per day. Thereafter, the number of feedings continued to increase, while volume remained fairly stable between 1500 and 2000 cc.

Contents of Tube-Feeding Diets

The majority of references discussing content of tube feedings state that feedings should "contain reasonable portions of all nutrients essential for adequate nutrition,"[1] should be "nutritionally adequate,"[35] or should be "a properly balanced diet."[29] Most of the formulas for tube feeding reviewed in nutrition texts and hospital diet manuals either met or exceeded the recommended daily dietary allowances published by the Food and Nutrition Board. The usual caloric density of tube feeding diets is 1 cal per ml; Proudfit and Robinson have recommended 2000 cal per day.[35] Peaston indicated that increased calories, as well as increased protein, are needed in acute illness because of characteristic metabolic responses but did not state a recommended number of calories.[33] One source, discussing diet for patients on a neurological service, recommended a caloric intake of 2000 to 2500 for tube-fed patients.[28] Pareira recommended 3500 or more cal per day for the rehabilitation of nutritionally debilitated patients.[32]

In this study, 30 of a total 39 diets using tube feeding had a caloric density of 1 cal per ml. The caloric density ranged from 0.35 to 1.4 cal per ml. The mean 24-hour diet intake for the entire study period was 1318 ml with a standard deviation of 726 ml. Considering the mean diet intake in terms of calories per milliliter (1318 calories), it becomes evident that most patients in this study were not receiving the recommended daily caloric intake for patients fed by tube.

There are wide variations in the ratio of protein, carbohydrate, and fat content of diets recommended both in nutrition textbooks and in journal articles for tube feedings. All of the variations shown

Table 11
Recommended Distribution of Substrates in Diets for Tube Feeding per 24 Hr.

SUBSTRATES (GM)	A (1)*	B (1)	C (28)	D (45)	E (25)
Protein	100	84	164	114	118
Fat	92	110	69	72	18
Carbohydrate	212	188	276	232	323

* Numbers in parentheses refer to references list.

in Table 11 are blenderized tube-feeding diets with the exception of Diet B, which is a milk-based formula. Diet C is a nonlactose diet; it is labeled high protein by its authors and is recommended to provide excess of protein for a debilitated and immobile patient in an effort to avoid bed sores.[28] One author recommended 150 gm of protein per day for tube feedings for "sick and injured patients."[32] Another stated that "in many circumstances, use of high protein feedings seems related to the myth that large quantities of dietary protein necessarily produce a superior nutritional result," but that "in the absence of protein deficit and internal environment consistent with nitrogen storage, protein intake above certain limits (1 gm per kg of body weight) is used chiefly as a source of calories and is converted to urea."[14] Thus, a high-protein tube-feeding diet can predispose to tube-feeding syndrome and dehydration.

Only one source reviewed stated limitations for protein–fat–carbohydrate ratios in tube-feeding diets.[23] Kee recommended a carbohydrate intake for 24 hours not exceeding 150 gm and proteins and fats of not more than 120 gm, and stated that diets with higher concentrations caused diarrhea or nausea.

The diets used in this study contained a wide variation in the ratio of protein, carbohydrate, and fat content. In Table 12 are five

Table 12
Distribution of Substrates in Five Study Diets

SUBSTRATES* (GM)	DIET IDENTIFICATION NO.				
	20	*25*	*30*	*51*	*77*
Protein	114	96	122	101	92
Fat	44	116	56	104	82
Carbohydrate	260	154	280	250	210

* Calculated for 2000 cal/24-hr intake.

of the diets administered on approximately 40 percent of the study days in this survey. Their protein, fat, and carbohydrate content was approximated to a 1300-cal diet, the mean caloric intake for this study. Diet 20 was the one used most frequently, representing 24 percent or 433 days and administered to 38 patients. On the basis of a 1300-cal intake, the patients on Diet 20 received carbohydrate content that exceeds recommended amounts for a 24-hour period, protein content sufficient for a 70-kg patient without predisposing to tube-feeding syndrome, and a low fat intake.

PATIENT RESPONSE TO TUBE FEEDING

Gastrointestinal Responses

Changes in stool frequency and consistency are among the most frequently reported responses to nasogastric tube feeding. In addition, abdominal cramps, stomach distention, nausea, vomiting, constipation, and diarrhea have been noted. Of these, diarrhea has been identified as the most common complication in both textbooks, [4,29,9,25,27,45,46] and journals.[10,16,17,23,8] However, the incidence of diarrhea is rarely identified, and when reports appear, they are somewhat conflicting. Pareira reported that only 7 percent of the 320 patients he studied developed diarrhea, and of these, 5 percent had mild diarrhea that was stopped by slowing the rate of feeding. Only 2 percent suffered from severe and continued diarrhea.[32] Unfortunately, in this study as well as in the following studies, the definition of diarrhea was either vague or nonexistent. Metzmeier and McDowell reported that diarrhea afflicted less than 1 percent of the patients when formula designed to overcome diarrhea was used.[28] The new formula differed from the old formula in that "it uses no milk and includes pureed vegetables and meat which add bulk to the intestinal contents." No statistics were included to indicate the incidence of diarrhea with the old formula. Jones and Peaston identified a 20-percent incidence of diarrhea in a group of severely ill patients who were on controlled ventilation for a variety of disorders.[22] The diet used in tube feeding contained Complan—a milk powder—and lactose. The diarrhea was severe and sometimes fatal, and the cause, according to Jones and Peaston, was unlikely to be hyperosmolarity, as evidenced by laboratory studies of the patients. Two adjustments in the tube feeding were made: lactose was replaced with glucose, and roughage in the form of methylcellulose was added. With these changes, diarrhea was reduced to less than 5 percent.

Several causes for diarrhea were identified in the literature. Osmotic diarrhea can be caused by an over-rich mixture,[23] or one in which the carbohydrate is too concentrated.[45] Such mixtures may result when prepared feedings are used for high-calorie feeding; for example, if a 3000-calorie tube feeding was ordered and Sustagen alone was used, the feeding would provide 180 grams of protein, 500 grams of carbohydrate, and 30 grams of fat. For such a high-calorie diet, Williams recommended combining Sustagen with enough blenderized tube-feeding formula to keep the carbohydrate down to 340 grams.[45] Mitchell et al. defined an over-rich formula as one containing too much fat, and recommended decreasing the fat content in order to control diarrhea.[29]

Gormican identified the introduction of cold tube feeding as causing diarrhea; thus he recommended the administration of warmed tube feedings.[16] The temperature of the cold feedings was not identified. In conflict with Gormican's idea, is the Holt study, which found no difficulty when feeding cold formula to infants.[20] Fason recommended refrigerated formula to prevent bacterial growth and found no ill effects from low temperature of administration.[11]

Diarrhea has been caused by milk-based formulas.[28,41] It has been explained on the basis of a suggested relative deficiency in lactase in adults. Other causes include contamination of the formula by coliform bacteria and staphylococci, [23,27] Salmonella infection from the use of raw eggs,[29] and parasitic disease from the use of uncooked meat.[13] Spoilage of the feeding in the tube from inadequate washing of the tube following administration of a feeding is another cause of diarrhea suggested by Metheny and Sniveley.[27] Two other possible causes less frequently cited include too-rapid administration of cold formula,[31] and a lack of bulk and fruit pectin in a usual diet.[29] It is apparent from this review that the incidence and causes of diarrhea vary greatly and may be related to a number of different aspects of the procedure of tube feeding and diet.

In this study, stool frequency of patients was reported on 1427 of the 1730 study days. The data revealed that no stool was passed on 44 percent of the study days, and one stool occurred on 31 percent of the study days. Fourteen percent of the patients had three or more stools per day for the 20-day study period. The percentage of patients reporting no stool showed a trend by study day, so that although a large proportion of patients showed no stool on the first and second days of the study period, the stool frequency thereafter remained fairly consistent, with about 35 to 40 percent of patients reporting no stool. A positive correlation was noted between the number of feedings per day and the number of stools (Pearson *r*; $p < .001$). There was also a positive correlation with $p < .001$ between total liquid diet taken daily and the number of stools per day. These findings are, of course, associated with several factors, including an increase in waste products, greater water content of stool, and more frequent stimulation of peristalsis by frequent meals. When the rate of administration of feeding was compared with the number of stools per day, there was a positive correlation ($r = .406$). The specific effects of frequency, rate, and volume per feeding, and their causal relationship to stool frequency will be examined in future studies.

Stool Consistency

Stool frequency alone cannot be considered the criterion for diarrhea or constipation but must be considered in conjunction with the consistency of the stool. Stool consistency in this study was rated on a nine-point scale from watery to hard and dry. The average consistency of stools was recorded for each day. Stool-consistency data were described on 626 of the 1730 study days. It is likely that consistency of stool would be more likely to be reported when it was something "unusual," i.e., when it was either too loose or too hard and dry. Thus, these data are taken only as indicative and are not considered definitive in terms of stool consistency with tube feedings. During the study period, more watery to soft, formed stools were reported than normal to hard, dry stools. Eighteen percent of the stools reported were liquid or creamy, and 22 percent were soft and formed. The percentage of stools reported for each type of stool consistency is shown in Table 13. There was a high incidence of stools of softer or looser consistency. There was no correlation between the rate of administration of feedings and the consistency of stools. There was a significant positive relation between incidence of stools of softer consistency and the number of feedings per day ($p < .001$).

Nausea, Vomiting, and Other GI Distress

On 238 of the 744 periodic days when data related to patient responses were collected, 12 percent of the patient responses

Table 13
Incidence of Stool Consistency*

CONSISTENCY	STOOLS (%)
No Stool	9
Watery	8
Creamy, liquid	18
Loose, mushy	10
Loose, soft	13
Formed, with some liquid	2
Soft, formed	22
Normal, formed	8
Hard	8
Hard, dry	2

* N = 626 days.

were "nauseated." Vomiting was reported on 28 days. Its incidence did not vary with the length of time the patient had been receiving tube feedings, and it occurred until the end of the study period. It is not known if the tube placement, rate of feeding, adverse reaction to feeding, medication, or anxiety were associated with the incidences of nausea and vomiting. Belching was reported by five patients. In a pilot study of a small group of normal subjects receiving tube feedings, belching was a common occurrence, leading one to suspect that when this symptom was present, it was often not recorded.

On 7 percent of the periodic days, distention was reported. The degree of severity was not known. Thirty-five of the 44 reports of distention were from patients on bedrest. Borborygmus was reported on 16 periodic days. It was not known whether these symptoms were reported because of the distress they caused or whether they were response-elicited upon questioning by the investigators. Flatus was reported on 50 days; it was more frequent in patients on bedrest than in those on some ambulation.

As in this study, the literature, too, reports a variety of gastrointestinal complications in addition to diarrhea. Brunner et al. mentioned nausea and recommended decreasing the amount of feeding until the nausea decreases and then gradually increasing the feeding to the desired amount.[6] Fallis and Barron,[10] Gregg and Rees,[18] and Metheny and Snively[27] also advised decreasing the rate of tube-feeding administration when nausea occurred.

Phipps and Barker stated that abdominal distention can be prevented by administering tube feeding at cold or room temperature, implying that warmed feedings cause the stomach to distend.[34] Metheny and Snively also noted occurrence of abdominal distention and excessive peristalsis and recommended giving the feeding slowly to prevent distention.[27] Shafer et al. cautioned against overfilling (more than 100 to 200 milliliters within 2 to 3 hours) and stated that it can cause vomiting and aspiration.[37] Only one reference referred to gastric bleeding as a complication, and there was no indication of the incidence or cause of such bleeding.[27]

Weight Change During Tube Feeding

Few references were found in the literature to patients' weight in relation to tube feeding. Taylor described a group of patients, weighed three times a week, who usually had gained weight while being fed by tube.[40] Data on the number of subjects and the amount of weight gained were not provided. In Pareira's study, success of tube feeding was established in most patients by an increase in weight gain as well as by positive nitrogen balance and an increase in the hemoglobin and plasma protein concentrations.[32]

Weights of 36 of the 121 patients in this study were recorded prior to the initiation of feeding and at intervals during feeding. Eleven patients gained an average of 5.9 pounds and 21 lost an average of 7.1 pounds during the study period of up to 20 days. Four patients' weights remained the same. During the second week of tube feedings, more subjects lost weight than gained weight.[13,6]

Changes in Fluid and Electrolyte Balance and Hematologic Values

Several complications of tube feedings that affect the fluid and electrolyte balance in the body have been identified. Gault reported severe dehydration and hypernatremia associated with high-protein feedings.[14] In an extended analysis of 3 patients and a comparison with 13 other patients with hypernatremia associated with tube feeding of high protein, Gault contended that patients who are unconscious or who because of concomitant problems (tracheostomy) cannot communicate or alleviate their thirst can rapidly develop the tube-feeding syndrome of hypernatremia, azotemia, and dehydration. The time course of the development of this syndrome is illustrated by a case described by Walike.[42] This complication is most likely to occur in patients whose fluid losses are increased (i.e., diarrhea) and where water-protein ratios in tube feeding are higher than those ordinarily well tolerated. Patients with potentially impaired renal function are also prone to the development of tube-feeding syndrome.

Ohlson[31] and Day and Buckell[8] referred to the danger of protein or salt overload with tube feeding and advised monitoring of the patient's urine solute concentration, BUN, electrolytes, and hemoglobin. Day and Bucknell identified the need for careful monitoring of the unconscious tube-fed patient who cannot react to thirst.[8] They described a tube-fed patient who regained consciousness after the feeding was modified to overcome the solute overload. Kee indicated that the usual ratio of 1 calorie per cc may not be adequate to provide sufficient water for a patient on a high-protein diet.[23]

The present study found that 1 cal per cc was the most common diet formulation; however, no cases of frank tube-feeding syndrome were observed in this sample. Over the total study days there were 80 elevated BUNs reported for 25 percent of the patients (31 patients). Thirty-five percent of these elevations fell into the 63 to 92 mg percent range noted by Gault to be marked with azotemia associated with tube-feeding syndrome.[14] Approximately 46 percent of the 80 incidents were in the 20 to 39 mg percent range (slightly elevated). Unimproved or decreasing consciousness levels and thirst were reported in less than 10 percent of the patients. Hematocrits showed increases of 10 percent in 6 patients and decreases of 6 to 11 percent in 8 patients. Case analyses of these results could produce some indication of diet-related hematologic changes.

Attitudes and Adjustment to Tube Feedings

The normal process of food intake involves an intermingling of interpersonal and emotional experiences as well as physiological and psychological factors.[7,15] For example, fear can slow down peristaltic action, whereas anger and hostility can speed it up. Unfortunately, many gaps exist in the understanding of such interplay.[15]

The procedure of tube feeding represents a drastic change in the physical conditions of food and food intake. For these reasons, patients' attitudes toward and adjustment to the procedure must be affected by it. Mitchell et al. stated that most patients found it difficult to accept tube feedings.[29] Nurses play a decisive role in the adjustment a patient makes to the procedure. Smith stated that the nursing care of the patient being fed by tube can be easy or difficult—pleasant for the patient or untidy and distressing.[38] The outcome depends to a large extent on the nurse's attitude and her appreciation of the patient's feelings.

Unfortunately, very little is known about patient attitudes or feelings with regard to tube feeding. This study found only scant information on the medical records relating to these responses. Little was known about the emotional status of tube-fed patients, with the exception of the presence of "some" or "extreme" nervousness on 51 percent of the days. Patients were asked about their sensations and perception relating to tube feedings. No preferences were expressed concerning the temperature of the feedings. On 39 study days, complaints of fullness were recorded, with two-thirds of these complaints subsequently resulting in refusals of one or more feedings. It is apparent from the scarcity of information in the literature and from this study that we need to learn more about patient attitudes and adjustment to tube feedings.

SUMMARY

This study has attempted to provide an overview of patients receiving tube feeding—their characteristics, their responses, and methods of feeding them. Current practices of tube feedings were described. Where noted on the hospital records, patients' responses to these tube feedings were described. It is apparent from the large-scale literature survey that very little is known about the scientific bases and rationale for much of current practice concerning both the methods and diet types used in the procedure. Even less is known about the psychological effects and the nursing measures that might be used to improve this area of patient response. This study has documented the need for much additional research on tube feedings and the effects on people. The investigators are currently initiating studies to improve the success of tube feedings by determining the function of several variables in patient responses to tube feeding. Included as variables in those projected studies are: lactose versus nonlactose diets; osmolality of diets; rate, volume, and frequency of diet administration; location of the feeding tube; and nursing interventions to reduce patient stress.

REFERENCES

1. Anderson, L. et al. *Nutrition in nursing.* Philadelphia: Lippincott, 1972.
2. Barron J. Tube feeding of postoperative patients. *Surgical Clinics of North America,* 1959, *39,* 1481–1491.
3. Barron, J., Prendegast, J. J., Jocz, M. W. Food pump: New approach to tube feeding. *Journal of the American Medical Association,* 1956, *161,* 621–622.
4. Beland, I. L. *Clinical nursing: Pathophysiological and psychosocial approaches* (2d ed.). New York: Macmillan, 1970.
5. Bouchard, R. *Nursing care for the cancer patient.* St. Louis: Mosby, 1967.
6. Brunner, L. S. et al. *Textbook of medical–surgical nursing.* Philadelphia: Lippincott, 1970.
7. Brusch, H. *Eating disorders.* New York: Basic Books, 1973.
8. Day, S., Buckell, M. Feeding the unconscious patient. *Proceedings of the Nutrition Society,* 1971, *30,* 184–190.
9. DuGas, B. W. *Kozier and DuGas introduction to patient care: A comprehensive approach to nursing* (2d ed.). Philadelphia: W. B. Saunders, 1972.
10. Fallis, L. S. & Barron, J. Gastric and jejunal alimentation with fine polyethylene tubes. *Archives of Surgery,* 1952, *65,* 373.
11. Fason, M. F. Controlling bacterial growth in tube feedings. *American Journal of Nursing,* 1967, *67,* 1246–1247.
12. Fuerst, E. V. & Wolff, L. *Fundamentals of nursing.* Philadelphia: Lippincott, 1969.
13. Garb, S. *Essentials of therapeutic nutrition.* Philadelphia: Springer, 1958.
14. Gault, H. M. et al. Hypernatremia, azotemia, and dehydration due to high-protein tube feeding. *Annals of Internal Medicine,* 1968, *68, 778–791.*
15. Giller, H. L. et al. Self-medication programs in public hospitals. I. A survey of practices in veterans administration hospitals. *Hospital and Community Psychiatry,* 1966, *17,* 355–356.
16. Gormican, A. Prepackaged tube feedings. *Hospitals,* 1970, *44,* 58–60.
17. Gormican, A., & Liddy, E. Nasogastric tube feedings. *Postgraduate Medicine,* 1973, *53,* 71–76.
18. Gregg, S. H., & Rees, O. M. *Scientific principles in nursing.* St. Louis: Mosby, 1970.
19. Hanson, R. L. Effects of administration of cold and warmed tube feedings. In M. V. Batey (ed.), *Communicating nursing research.* Boulder, Colo.: WICHE, 1973.

20. Holt, E. et al. A study of premature infants fed cold formulas. *Journal of Pediatrics,* 1964, *61,* 556–561.
21. Horsch, D. A cost analysis of tube-feeding procedures. *Hospitals,* 1966, *40,* 97–101.
22. Jones, E. S., & Peaston, M.J.T. Metabolic care during acute illness. *Practitioner,* 1966, *196,* 271.
23. Kee, J. Fluid imbalance in elderly patients *Nursing,* 1973, *3,* 40–43.
24. Kozier, B. B., & DuGas, B. W. *Fundamentals of patient care.* Philadelphia: W. B. Saunders, 1967.
25. Krause, M. *Food, nutrition, and diet therapy* (4th ed.). Philadelphia: W. B. Saunders, 1966.
26. Matheney, R. V., Nolan R., Ehrhart, A., & Griffin, G. J. *Fundamentals of patient-centered nursing.* St. Louis: Mosby, 1968.
27. Metheny, N. M., & Snively, W. D., Jr. *Nurses' handbook of fluid balance.* Philadelphia: Lippincott, 1967.
28. Metzmeier, C., & McDowell, S. New formula for tube feeding. *New York State Journal of Medicine,* 1961, *61,* 2061–2064.
29. Mitchell, H. S. et al. *Cooper's nutrition in health and disease* (15th ed.). Philadelphia: Lippincott, 1968.
30. Noyes, A., Camp, W., & van Sickel, M. *Psychiatric nursing* (6th ed.). New York: Macmillan, 1964.
31. Ohlson, M., ed. *Handbook of experimental and therapeutic diets.* Philadelphia: Burgess, 1962.
32. Pareira, M. D. *Therapeutic nutrition with tube feeding.* Springfield: C. C. Thomas, 1959.
33. Peaston, M.J.T. External metabolic balance studies during nasogastric feeding in serious illnesses requiring intensive care. *British Medical Journal,* 1966, *2,* 1367–1368.
34. Phipps, W., & Barker, W. L. Respiratory insufficiency and failure. In Lawrence Metgler et al. (Eds.) *Concepts and practices of intensive care for nurse specialists.* Philadelphia: Charles Press, 1969.
35. Proudfit, F. T. & Robinson, C. H. *Normal and therapeutic nutrition* (12th ed.). New York: Macmillan, 1961.
36. Saunders, W. H., Havener, W. H., Fair, C. J., & Hickey, J. *Nursing Care in eye, ear, nose and throat disorders* (2d ed.). St. Louis: Mosby, 1968.
37. Shafer, K. N. et al. *Medical–surgical nursing.* St. Louis: Mosby, 1967.
38. Smith, A. V. Nasogastric tube feeding. *American Journal of Nursing,* 1957, *57,* 1451–1452.
39. Sutton, A. I. *Bedside nursing techniques in medicine and surgery* (2d ed.). Philadelphia: W. B. Saunders, 1969.

40. Taylor, B. F. Taking food and fluids through a tube. *American Journal of Nursing,* 1953, *53,* 303.

41. Walike, B. C. & Walike, J. W. Lactose content of tube feeding diets as a cause of diarrhea. *Laryngoscope,* 1973, *83,* 1109–1115.

42. Walike, J. W. Tube feeding syndrome in head and neck surgery. *Archives of Otolaryngology,* 1969, *89,* 117–120.

43. White, D. T., Rubino, E., & De Lorey, P. D. *Fundamentals: The foundation of nursing.* Englewood Cliffs, N.J.: Prentice-Hall, 1972.

44. Williams, K. & Walike, B. Effect of temperature of tube feeding on gastric motility in monkeys. *Nursing Research,*1975, *24,* 4–9.

45. Williams, S. R. *Nutrition and diet therapy* (2d ed.). St. Louis: Mosby, 1973.

46. Wohl, M. G. Principles of dietotherapy. In M. G. Wohl and R. S. Goodhart (Eds.) *Modern Nutrition in Health and Disease* (4th ed.). Philadelphia: Lea & Febiger, 1970.

LACTOSE CONTENT OF TUBE-FEEDING DIETS AS A CAUSE OF DIARRHEA*

Barbara Caleen Walike, Ph.D., and Joseph W. Walike, M.D.

ABSTRACT

Tube feedings are frequently used by otolaryngologists in treating head and neck malignancies and other diseases. Common side effects of these diets include: borborygmi, meteorism, cramping, distention and diarrhea. These may vary from mild gastrointestinal distress to incapacitating diarrhea. This study investigated the role of lactose as a possible cause of diarrhea associated with tube-feeding diets. Lactose, the primary carbohydrate of milk, is the basic ingredient of most tube feeding diets.

Two identical diets, differing only in the presence or absence of 7 percent lactose, were administered to 11 patients in a double blind fashion. Each diet was given to each patient for approximately 10 consecutive days. The patients were studied in clinical research units where meticulous intake and output and total nitrogen balance studies were possible.

Nine of the 11 patients had a significant increase in the frequency of stools and a shift toward a more liquid stool consistency while on the lactose containing diet. Only two of these nine patients revealed a classical intolerance to lactose as indicated by a flat lactose tolerance test. The remaining seven patients had a relative lactose intolerance. This was clinically apparent only when they ingested a large quantity of lactose such as is contained in the usual tube-feeding diet.

---

*Presented at the Meeting of the Western Section of the American Laryngological, Rhinological, and Otological Society, Inc., Pebble Beach, Calif., February 4, 1973. From the Departments of Physiological Nursing, Physiology and Biophysics (B.C.W.), and Otolaryngology (J.W.W.), University of Washington, Seattle, Washington. This study was supported by NIH Grants: GCRCB-RR-37, (University Hospital), RR-133 (Harborview Medical Center), and NU00369 (University of Washington), Ross Laboratories, and the Northwest Medical Research Foundation, Inc.

We acknowledge the excellent assistance in data collection by the staff of the Clinical Research Units and by Mrs. Joanne Marshall and Mrs. Diane Clowers.

Reprinted with permission from Walike, B. C. & Walike, J. W. Lactose content of tube-feeding diets as a cause of diarrhea. The Laryngoscope, 1973, 83, 1109–1115.

Because lactose is not necessary for adequate nutrition, these data suggest that its elimination in tube-feeding diets would result in more comfortable and efficient tube feeding.

INTRODUCTION

The relative simplicity and safety of nasogastric tube feeding tends to obscure its high incidence of side effects and complications. Among the most common problems encountered are gastrointestinal distress, borborygmi, meteorism, cramping, and diarrhea. Such disturbances can cause or contribute to excoriation, discomfort, and generally retarded postoperative progress. Even the sometimes dire complication of tube-feeding syndrome involving dehydration, hypernatremia, hyperchloremia, and azotemia[1] may be initiated or exacerbated by diarrhea.

The suggested causes of this diarrhea include: rate of administration of the tube feeding, temperature of the liquid diet, location of the tube tip, osmolality of the diet, and contents of the diet. While each of these may contribute to the incidence of diarrhea with tube feedings, no cause and effect relationship has been demonstrated, and no prescriptions have been declared to reduce or eliminate this complication.

The present study focused upon the unique content of tube-feeding diets as a potential cause of gastrointestinal symptoms. While the specific ingredients of the liquid diets used for tube feedings vary widely, milk is one nutrient common to almost all preparations. Milk is the usual basis for both hospital-formulated and commercial tube-feeding diets.

Intolerance to milk, or more specifically, to its principle carbohydrate—lactose—is known to cause diarrhea and other gastrointestinal complaints.[2,3,4] Lactose intolerance occurs when an insufficient amount of the enzyme, lactase, is present in the brush border of the mucosa of the jejunum.[5,6] Lactase is required to split the disaccharide, lactose, into its component monosaccharides, glucose and galactose, which are absorbed in the small intestine. With lactase deficiency, the unsplit lactose passes into the large intestine where it apparently acts by two methods to produce diarrhea. It exerts an osmotic force in the colon, thus drawing fluids into the lumen, and the lactose is fermented by bacteria into organic acids which act as irritants to the mucosa of the large intestine.

The results are cramping, gas production, borborygmi, and diarrhea.

Three types of lactose intolerance have been described:[7] (1) congenital lactose intolerance or lactase deficiency is a relatively rare condition producing severe diarrhea in neonates; (2) secondary lactase deficiency can be seen following many diseases which affect the small intestinal mucosa and its brush border, particularly sprue and acute infectious diarrhea; and (3) acquired lactase deficiency is seen in patients who tolerated milk well as infants but later developed intolerance. It is this third type of lactose intolerance which probably is important in the diarrhea frequently associated with tube feedings.

Three methods are used to detect lactose-intolerant patients: (1) the lactose tolerance test (LTT) consisting of the oral administration of 50 or 100 gm lactose (or 2 gm/kg) and the subsequent monitoring of blood glucose as in the glucose tolerance test. A rise of less than 20–25 mg percent indicates lack of hydrolysis of lactose due to lactase deficiency; (2) symptoms of intolerance, including gas, cramping and/or diarrhea following the LTT or the ingestion of milk; and (3) a peroral or surgically obtained biopsy of the jejunal mucosa showing a deficiency of the lactase.

During the last 10 years much interest has been focused upon the incidence and etiology of this acquired enzyme defect.[8] It has been demonstrated that lactose intolerance is present in almost all adult nonhuman mammals and in most of the world's people, with only a few exceptions. Northern European Caucasians and their descendents, and a small number of Africans are the only groups in which lactose tolerance is widespread among adults. One study carried out in the United States found that 90–95 percent of the Negroes but only 5–10 percent of the Caucasians were lactase deficient.[9] It appears that adult tolerance of lactose is a genetic adaptation which evolved around an undetermined advantage conferred upon milk drinkers.

One might at this point conclude that lactose-free diets should be used for non-Caucasian patients, but that among Caucasians this would not be so important, due to the small percentage of intolerant adults. Clinically, however, it was our impression that diarrhea occurred in more than 5–10 percent of our Caucasian patients. The present study was designed to determine what proportion of the diarrhea of tube feeding could be accounted for by the lactose content of the diet, and what other factors might contribute to any remaining gastrointestinal symptoms.

METHODS

All patients included in this study had head and neck malignancies, with no history of gastrointestinal, renal, neurological, or endocrine disorders. All were in general good health except for cancer. Their postoperative course would normally require the use of nasogastric tube feedings. As soon as possible, patients were moved from intensive care units to the Clinical Research Units of either the University Hospital or Harborview Medical Center. The use of these research units made possible the detailed and complete recording of input and output data. Special forms were developed to provide uniformity in the collection of data and in the recording of stool frequency and consistency.

Two homogenized sterile liquid diets were specifically prepared for this study by a commercial laboratory. Both contained all of the required nutrients, vitamins, and minerals and had a caloric density of 1 kcal/cc. The diets were identical, with the exception that one contained 7 percent lactose while the other was lactose-free.* Both diets contained corn syrup solids; however, additional corn syrup solids were added to the lactose-free diet to make the two diets equivalent in caloric value.

Patients were placed on each of the two tube-feeding diets for 10 consecutive days. One-half of the group received the lactose diet first, then the nonlactose diet; the other half were given the diets in the reverse order. The order of the diets for each patient was not known to either the physicians or nurses involved in the patient care and data collection. The amount of intake was determined by the needs of each patient.

Complete laboratory data were obtained on each patient, including periodic determinations of electrolytes, serum osmolality, cholesterol, triglycerides, total protein, glucose and complete blood count. A glucose tolerance test and a lactose tolerance test were obtained on each patient at the conclusion of the study.

RESULTS

Eleven patients were studied for a mean of 9.4 days on each of the two diets. The average daily diet intake for the nine males was 2411 calories or ml, while the mean for the two females was

ENSURE™ by Ross Laboratories.

1945 calories. The intakes on the two diets did not differ significantly for each individual patient.

Both stool frequency and consistency showed marked differences between the two diet periods. In Figure 1 the ratios of the number of stools on the lactose containing diet to the number on the nonlactose diet are shown for the 11 patients. Most patients had two to four times more stools on the lactose-containing diet, with one patient having 12 times more stools. Only two patients showed no difference between the number of stools on the two diets. These two were labeled tolerant, while the nine who showed more frequent stools on the lactose-containing diet were labeled intolerant.

The consistency of stools differed markedly between the two diets, as shown in Figure 2. The average stool consistency for each of the 11 patients on each diet is indicated. The stools were looser and more liquid during the period on the lactose containing diet.

The results of the lactose tolerance tests for all patients are summarized in Figures 3 and 4. Figure 3 reveals the peak rise of blood glucose for each patient during the LTT. As in Figure 1, the

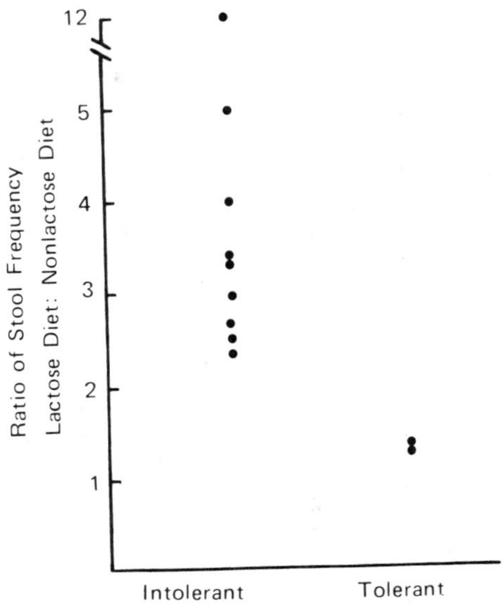

Fig. 1. Comparison of stool frequency on lactose-containing and nonlactose diets. Two patients had approximately the same number of stools on each diet and are labeled "tolerant." All others had at least twice as many stools on the lactose diet and are labeled "intolerant."

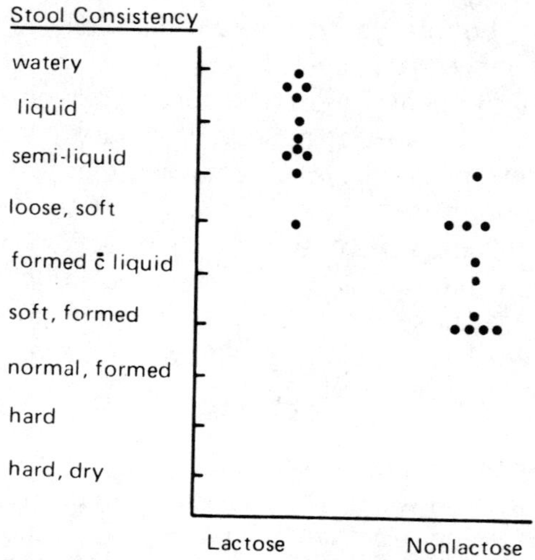

Fig. 2. Comparison of stool consistency on lactose-containing and nonlactose diets. The usual consistency for each of the 11 patients on each diet is indicated by a dot.

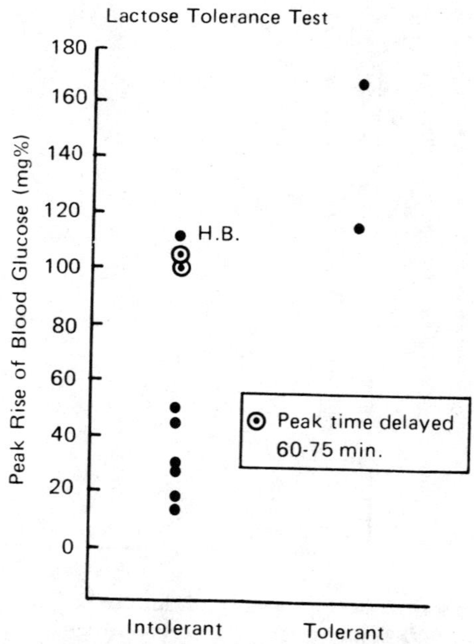

Fig. 3. Peak rise of blood glucose during lactose tolerance test. Patients are separated into tolerant and intolerant as in Fig. 1. Details are discussed in text.

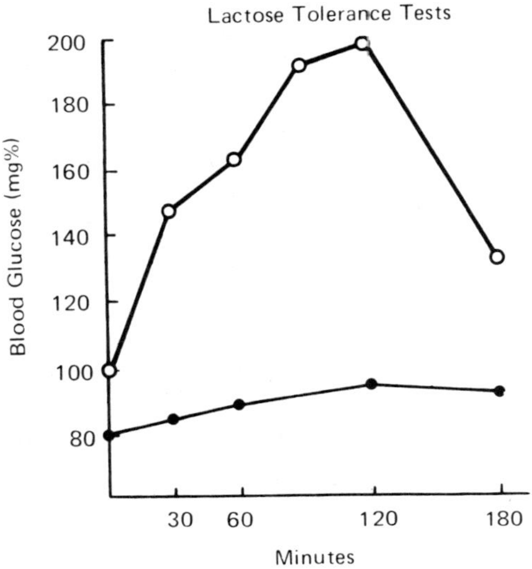

Fig. 4. Lactose tolerance tests for two "intolerant" patients. Lower curve is flat, showing classical response of lactose intolerant patient. The upper curve shows the delayed peak rise which was seen in two patients with a relative intolerance to lactose.

patients in Figure 3 are divided into intolerant and tolerant, according to their stool-frequency ratios. Of the nine patients showing increased stool frequency on the lactose-containing diet, only two demonstrated the LTT curve which is classical for lactose intolerance. The curve for one of these patients is illustrated in Figure 4 and demonstrates a blood glucose rise of less than 20 mg percent.

How can one explain the seemingly normal peak rises of greater than 20 mg percent following LTT in the other 7 patients who were labeled clinically intolerant by their increased stool frequency on the lactose-containing diet? While these remaining 7 patients were able to hydrolyze some lactose, as indicated by the rises in blood glucose, it is our hypothesis that these patients have a relative deficiency of lactase. This deficiency, while permitting a reasonable rise of blood glucose following oral lactose, prevents the complete hydrolysis of the lactose load. It appears that even relatively small amounts of unhydrolyzed lactose, when passed into the large intestine, can cause increased frequency and more watery stools.

The presence of a relative deficiency of lactase in these patients is further supported by examination of the tolerance tests of the three intolerant patients who, nevertheless, showed high rises of blood glucose during the LTT. One of these patients (H. B.) had a blood glucose rise of 110 mg percent following oral lactose; however, an identically administered oral glucose load produced a significantly higher peak rise of 160 mg percent. Perhaps this difference between the peak glucose rises of the LTT and GTT represents an incomplete hydrolysis of lactose. Two patients, whose peak glucose rises are indicated by an encircled dot in Figure 3, differed from the other patients in that the time of their maximum rise following the lactose load was 60 to 75 minutes later than their respective peak rises following a glucose load; thus, these data also suggest a relative deficiency of lactase permitting the delayed and probably incomplete splitting of lactose. The complete LTT curve for one of these patients is shown in Figure 4.

CONCLUSIONS

1. The lactose content of liquid diets commonly used for nasogastric tube feedings is a major cause of diarrhea and other gastrointestinal disturbances.

2. The lactose tolerance test distinguished only 2 of the 9 patients who demonstrated increased stool frequency on the lactose-containing diet. It is, therefore, not an adequate test for determining the need for a lactose-free diet in tube-feeding patients.

3. A relative lactose intolerance, or the inability to utilize completely a large load of lactose, is probably present in the great majority of adults, even those with lactose tolerance test results which are considered normal.

4. Such a relative lactose intolerance will be clinically unimportant except under conditions where the size of the load of lactose challenges the patient's ability to hydrolyze the lactose. This lactase deficiency may become clinically significant where large amounts of lactose are included in the diet as is common for tube-fed patients. Lactose content may also be a significant cause of gastrointestinal disturbance in adult patients who ingest large quantities of milk, for example, ulcer patients or pregnant women. These groups of patients have not yet been studied.

5. The elimination of lactose from tube-feeding diets will reduce the gastrointestinal side effects of these diets.

REFERENCES

1. Walike, J. W. Tube-feeding syndrome in head and neck surgery. *Archives of Otolaryngology,* 1969, *89,* 533–536.
2. Cuatrecasas, P., Lockwood, D. H., & Caldwell, J. R. Lactase deficiency in the adult. *Lancet,* 1965, *1,* 14–18.
3. Jussila, J., Launiala, K., & Gorbatow, O. Lactase deficiency and a lactose-free diet in patients with "unspecific abdominal complaints." *Acta Medica Scandinavica,* 1969, *186,* 217–222.
4. Gudmand-Høyer, E, Dahlqvist, A., & Jarnum, S. The clinical significance of lactose malabsorption. *American Journal of Gastroenterology,* 1970, *53,* 460–473.
5. Dahlqvist, A., et al. Intestinal lactase deficiency and lactose intolerance in adults. *Gastroenterology,* 1963, *45,* 488–491.
6. McMichael, H. B., Webb, J., & Dawson, A. M. Jejunal disaccharidases and some obvations on the cause of lactase deciency. *British Medical Journal,* 1966, *2,* 1037–1041.
7. Alpers, D. H., & Isselbacher, K. J. Disaccharidase deficiency. *Advances in Metabolic Disorders,* 1970, *4,* 75–122.
8. Simoons, F. J. Primary adult lactose intolerance and the milking habit: A problem in biological and cultural interrelations. *American Journal of Digestive Diseases,* 1969, *14,* 819–836.
9. Bayless, T. M., & Rosensweig, N. S. A racial difference in the incidence of lactase deficiency. *Journal of the American Medical Association,* 1966, *197,* 968–972.

RELATIVE LACTOSE INTOLERANCE: A CLINICAL STUDY OF TUBE-FED PATIENTS*

Barbara C. Walike, Ph.D., Joseph W. Walike, M.D.

A relative intolerance of lactose was demonstrated in 14 of 16 patients receiving nasogastric tube feedings following surgery for head or neck carcinoma. Two liquid diets differing only in the presence or absence of lactose, were administered for 8 to 20 days per patient in a double-blind crossover study. Increased stool frequency, decreased stool consistency, and more frequent flatulence, borborygmi, and distention were found with the lactose diet, although classic lactose intolerance (plasma glucose rise of less than 26 mg/dl) was indicated in only 2 patients. Differences between amounts and times of peak rise following the glucose tolerance test and lactose tolerance test for each patient indicated the advisability of locating patients on a continuum of ability to hydrolyze lactose. The results indicate that lactose should be reduced or eliminated from tube-feeding diets to improve patient tolerance and comfort and to reduce diarrhea.(*JAMA* 238:948–951, 1977)

Lactose intolerance due to a deficiency of intestinal lactase has been well described and documented.[1,2] Its symptoms include diarrhea, abdominal cramps, fullness, flatulence, borborygmi, and nausea.[2] There have been many studies of lactose intolerance and of the complications of tube feedings, but none have dealt with

---

*From the Departments of Physiology, Biophysics, and Physiological Nursing (Dr B. Walike), and Otolaryngology (Dr J. Walike), University of Washington at Seattle, and the Mason Clinic, Seattle.

Dr B. Walike is now with the Department of Physiology, School of Medicine, University of Michigan, Ann Arbor.

Reprint requests to Department of Physiology, School of Medicine, University of Michigan, Ann Arbor, MI 48109 (Dr Hansen).

This investigation was supported by NIH grants NU00523 (University of Washington), RR-133 (Harborview Medical Center Clinical Research Unit), and NU00369 (University of Washington), and by Ross Laboratories and the Northwest Medical Research Foundation, Inc. A portion of this work was conducted through the Clinical Research Center Facility of the University of Washington supported by the National Institutes of Health (grant RR-37).

Margaret Heitkemper, MA, and Verlene Vanderburg supervised the data collection for this study. Lynne Kalnasy performed the statistical analyses and the data processing, and Terry Meijsen performed the stool analyses and nitrogen determinations.

one as a cause of the other. Yet the symptoms of lactose intolerance bear a striking similarity to the symptoms that are often associated with tube feedings: diarrhea, fullness, intolerance of or refusal to ingest adequate intakes, flatulence, borborygmi, nausea, and vomiting.

Lactose intolerance has been indicated by: (1) a peak rise in the blood glucose level of less than 20 or 26 mg/dl during a lactose tolerance test (LTT),[1] (2) gastrointestinal disturbance following either an LTT or consumption of milk,[2] (3) a lactase level below 2 IU/g wet mucosal weight or 10 IU/g protein as shown by intestinal biopsy specimens,[3] and (4) increased H_2 levels in breath analysis following lactose ingestion.[4] Some investigators require more than one of these indications for the diagnosis of lactose intolerance because measurements by these tests are highly variable and because the criteria for lactose malabsorption remain controversial.

Lactase deficiency has been demonstrated in 6 to 20 percent of white Americans and 60 percent of black Americans.[5] Several types of lactase deficiency have been described: (1) congenital lactase deficiency, a relatively rare condition that produces severe diarrhea in neonates, (2) secondary lactase deficiency, a reduction in lactase activity following many diseases that affect the mucosa of the small intestine, such as sprue, and (3) acquired lactase deficiency (also called primary lactase deficiency), a condition in which milk is not tolerated after weaning, in adolescence, or in adulthood.[4] The present study deals primarily with acquired lactase deficiency, which is often unknown and unsuspected. Persons with asymptomatic lactase deficiency can become symptomatic under three conditions: (1) lactase deficiency in combination with ulcerative or other gastrointestinal diseases where mucosal lesions result in further decrease of lactase, (2) increased lactose load, as in ulcer diets or milk-based formula diets, or (3) increased gastric emptying, as in postgastric resection.[5]

Milk-based formula diets are most commonly used for the tube feedings. Lactose generally constitutes 4 to 7 percent of these diets and as much as 22 percent in some liquid diets; it is also the major source of carbohydrates in commercially formulated diets. Therefore, an adequate caloric intake yields a lactose load of 80 to 210 g/24 hr, compared with the usual lactose intake by adult Americans of approximately 12 g per 240 ml glass of milk.[4] As little as 6 g of lactose can produce increased fluid in the lower small intestine of lactose intolerant patients, and as little as 3 g can cause symptoms.[6] Thus, the quantity of lactose in the tube-feeding formula that is clinically relevant can be extremely low for highly intolerant patients.

Patients receiving tube feedings containing lactose may suffer nutritional deficiencies owing to either limited intake because of discomfort, reduced absorption of nutrients, or H_2O soluble materials such as folic acid and iron.[6]

The present investigation demonstrated that lactose is frequently the cause of complications associated with tube feedings and showed that the LTT cannot always identify relative lactose intolerance.

MATERIALS AND METHODS

The subjects were 20 white patients (16 men, 4 women) ranging in age from 46 to 74 years, who were receiving nasogastric tube feedings after surgery for head and neck carcinoma. They had no history of gastrointestinal, renal, neurologic, or endocrine disorders, or milk intolerance. Fourteen patients were admitted to a clinical research unit where detailed metabolic determinations, including nitrogen balance studies and accurate assessment and analysis of intake and output, were carried out. The procedure of our study was explained to each patient, and written consent for participation was obtained.

For this study, a commercial laboratory prepared two sterile, homogenized formulas that were constituted to be as similar as possible. Both contained all required nutrients, vitamins, and minerals, and they had a caloric density of 1 kcal/cc. The two diets differed in that one contained lactose and the other did not. In the former, lactose was substituted for half of the carbohydrate or 7 percent by weight of the formula; this amounted to approximately 75 g lactose per liter of formula. The diets were coded to conceal their identity from the nursing, medical, and research staff, and the code was broken only after each patient had completed the study. Intake was calculated to meet the needs of each patient. The two diets were administered in random order so that half of the patients received the lactose-free diet initially. Eight of the patients were given each diet for 10 days, while the rest received each diet for successive periods of 4 to 9 days (total of 9 to 20 days per patient).

Periodic urine and stool analyses and blood chemistry determinations were run for each patient. The following protocol was used: liquid diet was administered at 2000 to 3000 kcal/day—6 feedings per day with the intake and code number of each can recorded; body weight was checked daily; blood sample levels of Na, K, Cl, CO_2, total protein, albumin, calcium, alkaline phosphatase, total bilirubin, BUN, glucose, creatinine, cholesterol, and osmolarity were checked on days 1, 3, 6, 8, 11, 13, 16, 18, and 21; 24-hour urine collections were analyzed for Na, K, Cl, creatinine, PO_4 and osmolarity; stool analyses included Na, K, percentage of fat, nitrogen, PO_4, percentage of ash, and wet and dry weight; glucose tolerance tests (GTTs) (100 g/250 ml H_2O) were done on day 21 with the following samples drawn: fasting, 15, 30, 60, 90, 120, 150, and 180 minutes; LTTs (100 g/250 ml H_2O) were done on day 22 using the same sampling times.

Blood chemistry, GTT, and LTT samples were determined by an autoanalyzer. An osmometer measured serum and urine osmolarity by freezing point. Sodium and potassium levels in urine and stool were determined with a flame photometer. Urine chloride, creatinine, and inorganic phosphate levels were measured by an autoanalyzer. Urine nitrogen and complete stool analyses were performed by the core Laboratory of the clinical research unit using the following methods: nitrogen analysis by the Kjeldahl method, stool phosphate analysis by the method of Kraml,[7] and stool fat content by the method of Roese-Gottlieb.[8]

RESULTS

Complete data were obtained from 16 patients; complications unrelated to tube feeding developed in 4 patients who then had to be removed from the study. Nitrogen balance and stool analysis was followed on 11 of the 16 patients.

Average caloric intake ranged from 1670 to 2880 kcal/day (mean, 2325 kcal/24 hr, 86.2 SEM). There was no important net gain or loss during the study, except for one patient who lost 2.0 kg on an average daily intake of 1830 kcal/24 hr. Nitrogen balance in the 11 patients ranged from +8.08 to −3.64 g/24 hr and averaged +1.92 g/24 hr (SEM, 1.1 g/24 hr). Between the two diet periods, there were no noticeable differences in nitrogen balance.

The caloric intakes of the two diets did not differ greatly between the two study periods, but most patients produced at least 1.5 times as many stools while receiving the lactose diet. The ratio of number of stools during the lactose diet period to the number

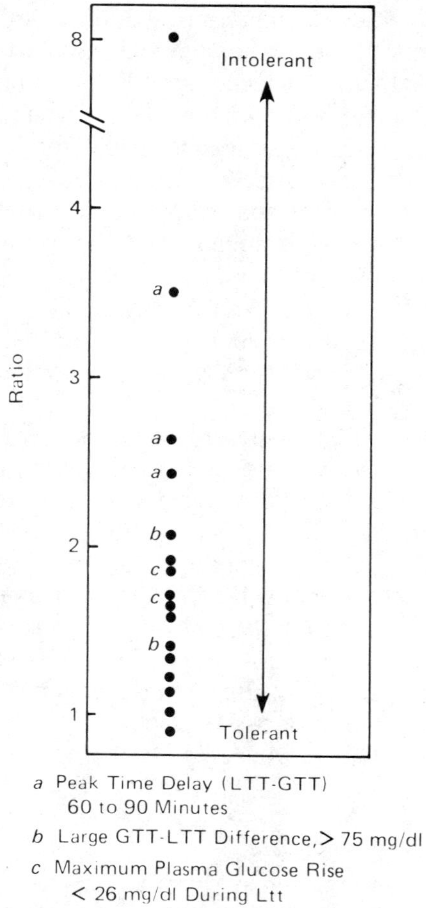

Fig. 1. **Ratio of number of stools during diet containing lactose to number of stools during lactose-free diet. Arrow indicates tolerance versus intolerance continuum. Specific patients are indicated by symbols for comparison of LTT-GTT results with stool frequencies on two diets.**

during the nonlactose diet period indicates that patients can be analyzed on a lactose tolerance–intolerance continuum (Figure 1). Stool consistency ranged from soft to hard when receiving the diet without lactose, but was predominantly loose to liquid when receiving the diet with lactose, as rated by nurse–clinicians and validated by stool ash analyses. The results of stool analyses are summarized in Table 1. Stool weight, percent water, and Na showed significant differences between the two diet periods.

The results of the LTT were viewed in relation to three values: (1) glucose rise above fasting during LTT, (2) peak glucose rise during GTT minus peak glucose rise during LTT, and (3) time of peak glucose rise during LTT with respect to peak rise during GTT. In only two patients (indicated by a small letter *c*, Figure 1) was classic lactase deficiency demonstrated by a plasma glucose rise of less than 26 mg/dl above fasting. While both were equally intolerant according to this criterion, they showed appreciable differences in the GTT peak rise minus LTT peak rise. One showed more symptoms while receiving the lactose diet and a large GTT-LTT peak rise difference (75 mg/dl).

Two other patients also demonstrated differences greater than 75 mg/dl between peak rises during GTT and LTT (indicated by a small *b*, Figure 1). These two also complained of gastrointestinal symptoms along with increased frequency of stools while receiving the lactose diet.

Three patients who showed otherwise normal LTT results had a peak time difference of 60 to 90 minutes between GTT and LTT glucose rise. These 3 patients (indicated by a small *a*, Figure 1) displayed an increase in stool frequency while receiving the lactose diet.

An example of one of these patient's stool frequency during the two diet periods and of his delayed LTT peak glucose rise with respect to his GTT glucose rise is shown in Figure 2. It is readily apparent that taken alone this patient's LTT would previously have been considered normal. However, these data indicating increased stool frequency, more severe symptoms, and delayed LTT peak

Table 1
Results of Stool Analyses*

	NONLACTOSE		LACTOSE		MEAN DIFFERENCE	SEM	*P* VALUE
	MEAN	SEM	MEAN	SEM			
Mean stool, weight/day	83.18	27.61	154.69	28.80	−71.51	26.79	.05
Water, %	82.87	0.88	86.14	0.81	−3.26	0.94	.01
Na, mEq/day	2.94	0.61	6.65	2.00	−3.71	1.58	.05
K, mEq/day	6.91	1.04	7.55	1.02	−0.64	1.10	NS
PO_4 g/day	0.67	0.10	0.64	0.06	0.03	0.12	NS
N, g/day	10.32	1.66	16.21	3.48	−5.89	2.86	NS
Fat, g/day	2.26	0.32	3.87	1.00	−1.61	1.02	NS

* Student's *t* test, n = 11.

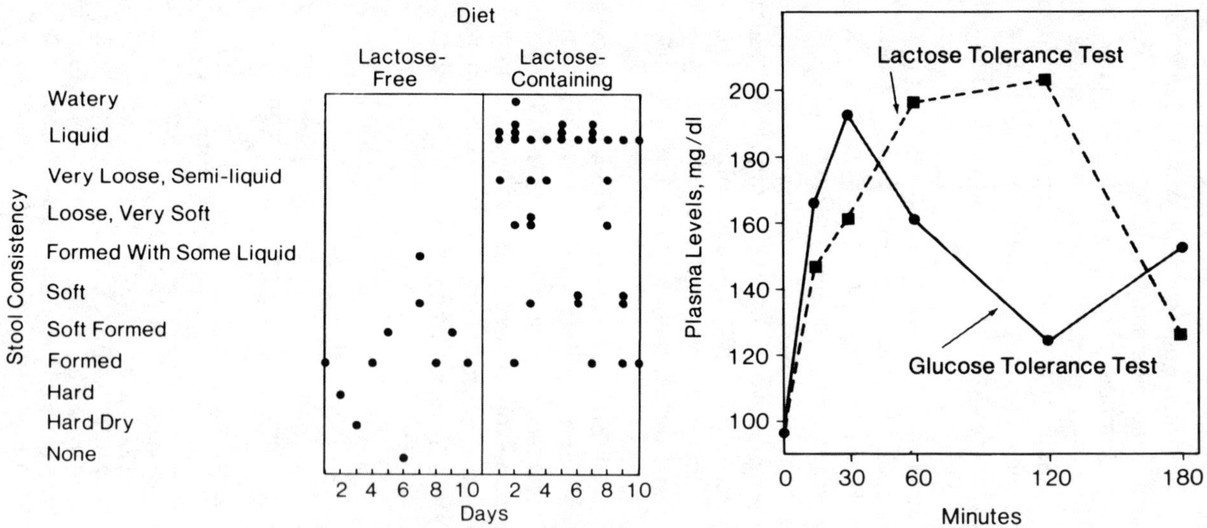

Fig. 2. *Left,* Comparison of stool frequencies and consistencies on two diets for patient 1. Each dot represents one stool (except for day 6 on lactose-free diet, in which there were no stools). Total number of stools during lactose-free diet period was 10 and total number of stools on lactose-containing diet was 35. *Right,* Results of glucose and lactose tolerance tests for patient 1.

rise clearly demonstrate that the cause of this patient's diarrhea was a relative intolerance of lactose.

During the lactose diet period, 9 patients complained of gastrointestinal distress, including flatulence, borborygmi, belching, nausea, and distention. Most patients experienced more than one symptom while receiving the lactose diet.

The levels of blood electrolytes, NA, K, Cl, CO_2, and Ca compared for the two study periods showed no significant changes. Urine Na and Cl were higher during the nonlactose diet period, and K, creatinine, PO_4, nitrogen, and volume levels showed no important differences.

COMMENT

The lactose content of a tube-feeding diet caused an increase in stool frequency and weight, a decrease in consistency, and increased gastrointestinal disturbances in 14 of 16 white patients with no history of intolerance to their normal consumption of milk. These changes were precipitated by unhydrolyzed lactose in the ileum and colon. Unhydrolyzed lactose increases the solute content and therefore the osmotic activity of the intestinal fluid and produces the following effects: (1) increased fluid load, particularly in the jejunum and ileum, (2) accelerated intestinal transit because of increased intraintestinal volume, (3) fermentation of lactose to lactic acid, which increases the solute content and may act as a bowel irritant, and (4) inadequate absorption of the fluid load presented to the colon. Since all other confounding variables were controlled, it is apparent that there was a relative insufficiency of intestinal lactase to handle the lactose load that accompanies most tube feedings. The existence of partial or relative lactose intolerance has been suggested.[2,3,5] Relative intolerance implies that under normal consumption the lactase level is sufficient, but when the lactose content is increased either by rapid gastric emptying or by increased lactose ingestion, the lactase is not adequate and symptoms become manifest. The majority of patients in this group clearly demonstrated intolerance when given the lactose-containing diet.

These results indicate limitations in the diagnostic value of the LTT, including the inadequacy of selecting an arbitrary level of plasma glucose rise for determining lactose intolerance. The LTT shows only severe cases of lactase deficiency, but does not indicate the existence of a relative deficiency. In our study, the difference in glucose rise was correlated with increased stool frequency and symptoms on lactose-containing diet in 3 patients who experienced peak LTT delay of 60 to 90 minutes, and in 3 other patients who demonstrated GTT-LTT differences of greater than 75 mg/dl. Although their glucose levels rose following lactose ingestion, the comparison between their symptomatic responses to the lactose-containing diet and the lactose and glucose tolerance tests suggests a relative intolerance to lactose or a slow and incomplete absorption of it.

CONCLUSION

On the basis of this study, we make three recommendations: (1) Reduce or eliminate lactose from the formulas of liquid diets to minimize diarrhea, distention, flatulence, fullness, and rejection of tube-feeding amounts needed for adequate intake. (2) Recognize that the usual arbitrary level of glucose rise (less than 26 mg/dl) is inadequate to indicate lactase deficiency. Both time of peak response and the amplitude of that response relative to a similarly administered GTT can greatly alter the interpretation of an LTT. (3) Consider lactose intolerance to be a relative phenomenon that must be defined by both the size of the lactose load and the total intestinal capacity to hydrolyze lactose.

REFERENCES

1. Newcomer, A., & McGill, D: Lactose tolerance tests in adults with normal lactase activity. *Gastroenterology,* 1966, *50,* 340–346.
2. Alpers, D., & Isselbacher, K.: Disaccharidase deficiency. *Adv. Metab. Disord.,* 1970, *4,* 75–122.
3. Pirk, F., & Skala, I.: Functional response of the digestive tract to the ingestion of milk in subjects suffering from lactose intolerance. *Digestion,* 1972, *5,* 89–99.
4. Calloway, O., & Chenoweth, W.: Utilization of nutrients in milk-and-wheat-based diets by men with inadequate and reduced abilities to absorb lactose: I. Energy and nitrogen. *Am. J. Clin. Nutr.,* 1971, *26,* 939–957.
5. Welsh, J. D., in discussion, Klotz, A. P., Lubos, M. C.: Gastrointestinal symptoms and intestinal lactase deficiencies: A word of caution. *Am. J. Dig. Dis.,* 1967, *12,* 424–425.

6. Bedine, M., & Bayless, T.: Intolerance of small amounts of lactose by individuals with low lactase levels. *Gastroenterology,* 1973, *65,* 735–743.

7. Kraml, M.: A semiautomated determination of phospholipids. *Clin. Chim. Acta,* 1966, *13,* 442–448.

8. Horowitz, W.: *Official Methods of Analysis of the Association of Official Analytical Chemists.* Association of Official Analytical Chemists, 1970, p 263.

APPENDICES

APPENDIX A

GUIDE TO READING RESEARCH CRITICALLY

Research Article/Report

Title and Author:

Journal in Which Reported:

Questions to be Considered

1. What was the problem that was studied?

2. Does this study help solve a clinical problem which you face currently? If so, describe the problem.

3. To what extent does the solution investigated in this study solve the clinical problem you have identified?

4. In what setting was the research conducted? Be specific and describe in detail (For example, was it in a laboratory or clinical setting? What type of institution? What type of unit? Was there anything about the setting that makes you think that it is not typical of clinical settings?)

5. In what ways is your practice setting similar or different from the setting in which the research was conducted?

6. What patients or clients were studied?
   a. primary diagnosis or condition
   b. sex
   c. age
   d. other

7. Is there anything about these patients or clients that makes you think they are atypical? How do they differ from the patients or clients you might involve in a trial of the research-based practice?

8. What was the total number of patients or clients studied? Is there any reason to question the adequacy of this number?

9. What is the independent variable that was studied? (An independent variable is the variable that comes first in time and is assumed to cause the effect that is being studied. It is often a nursing intervention, patient characteristic, or patient behavior that is studied to determine its effect.)

10. Is this independent variable a nursing intervention? If so, describe the intervention as it was carried out by the researcher.

11. What are the dependent variables in the study? (A dependent variable is the measured effect that is thought to result from, or depend on, the independent variable.)

12. How were these dependent variables measured in the study?

13. Which of these measurement methods are familiar to you? Which can be used in your setting?

14. What effects were seen in patients or clients that the author attributed to the independent variable (intervention)?

15. Do you agree that the independent variable (intervention) was responsible for the changes in patients/clients as stated by the author?

16. Based upon your knowledge and experience, what other rationale might explain the results of this study?

17. To what extent does the author discuss the reliability of the data collected? How was reliability achieved? At what level? (The concept of reliability suggests that if the measurement was repeated on the same patients, under the same conditions, the same results would be obtained.)

18. To what extent does the author discuss the validity of tools used in collecting the data? How was validity determined? (The concept of validity suggests that the instruments used to measure the effects of the interventions measure what they were supposed to measure.)

19. Does the author state that the conclusions reached are based on results that are statistically significant?

20. Based upon this report, can you ascertain whether or not the researcher has carried out other studies in this area? Does this study expand on prior research?

21. Are you familiar with other studies which address the same problem and/or the same intervention? How were the results similar or conflicting?

22. After critically examining this study, are you interested in using the intervention in your clinical practice? Why?

23. After reading this article, what additional information is needed to evaluate these findings.?

24. How would you go about obtaining the additional information if needed?

APPENDIX B

DEVELOPING RESEARCH-BASED INNOVATION PROTOCOLS: PROCESS, CRITERIA, AND ISSUES*

Karen B. Haller, Margaret A. Reynolds, and Jo Anne Horsley

The criteria and issues involved in a process of transferring research-based knowledge into innovation protocols for nursing practice are discussed. Three sets of criteria are identified: (a) criteria that pertain to evaluating and integrating studies that constitute a base, (b) criteria that address the issue of how relevant the base is for nursing practice, and (c) criteria related to the potential for evaluation in the clinical setting. The format of the innovation protocol is presented. It is suggested that the protocol may be seen as a form of methodological approximation between research and practice. It is also noted that the process involved in identifying research bases for utilization can serve to identify needs for the conduct of nursing research in the future.

---

*Ms. Karen B. Haller and Ms. Margaret A. Reynolds are doctoral students in clinical nursing research at the University of Michigan and research assistants for the Conduct and Utilization of Research in Nursing (CURN) Project. Dr. Jo Anne Horsley is professor of nursing at the University of Michigan School of Nursing and principal investigator of the CURN Project. Requests for reprints may be addressed to the CURN Project, School of Nursing, The University of Michigan, Ann Arbor, Michigan 48109. This paper was received August 10, 1978, was revised, and was accepted for publication February 15, 1979.

This research is supported by Division of Nursing, DHEW, Grant NU00542 awarded to the Michigan Nurses Association. The scientific work of the project is conducted by faculty and graduate students at the University of Michigan School of Nursing and the Institute for Social Research and at the Michigan State University School of Nursing.

This paper was presented under the title "Developing research-based practice innovations; Criteria, processes, and issues" at the Eleventh Annual Communicating Nursing Research Conference, Western Society for Research in Nursing, Portland, Oregon, May 4, 1978.

The authors acknowledge the contribution of Ms. Janet Bingle, former associate on the CURN Project, to early development of ideas embodied in this paper.

This paper deals with the criteria and issues involved in a process of transferring research-based knowledge into innovation protocols for nursing practice. Content for the paper developed from work on a funded project titled the Conduct and Utilization of Research in Nursing (CURN). Now in its fourth year of activity, CURN is addressing a widespread and critical problem in the nursing profession. The amount of sound nursing research has been increasing steadily, but often this research has had little appreciable impact on nursing practice (Aydelotte, 1976; Ketefian, 1975; Krueger, 1978). Project staff are investigating ways in which scientific knowledge may be transferred to the practice of nursing and ways in which clinical practice might influence nursing research so that it more closely approximates the clinical setting's methods and goals.

Requisite to this work is the identification and evaluation of nursing research that is suitable for transfer to practice settings. This process has involved retrieving, reviewing, and organizing studies into areas of conceptually related research, followed by an evaluation of each area's potential for use. The final step in this sequence is the development of "innovation protocols" for nursing care interventions based on the identified research. Although specific criteria have guided the process of transforming clinical research into such protocols. several issues of concern have emerged. It is our intent in this paper to describe the process and the criteria used and to delineate the issues that have arisen.

PROCESS

The project staff's experience with research utilization to date has demonstrated that considerable confusion exists among nurses regarding the differences between the conduct of research and the utilization of the knowledge resulting from such research. For example, when asked to describe how they might use research in their practice, nurses often cite a process of replication. It is important to differentiate the goals and, therefore, the people, knowledge, and context relevant for research conduct and research utilization, respectively. Research conduct is directed toward the production of knowledge that is generalizable beyond the population directly studied. The process of research utilization, on the other hand, is directed toward transferring specific research-based knowledge into actual practice. The conduct of research generally occurs in the academic context where people with specialized knowledge and skills in the methods of scientific inquiry can obtain the resources and control of conditions necessary. To be effective, however, research-based knowledge should be implemented and evaluated in a practice context where people with knowledge, skills, and experience in the methods of nursing practice can examine the relevance, means, and utility of new techniques (Horsley, Crane, & Bingle, 1978).

A key dimension on which the conduct of research varies from research utilization is methodology. The tenets of scientific methodology can be contrasted with those of the methodology of practice. Nurses in settings where research is conducted rely on scientific methodology that is systematic, controlled, and generally inflexible. Research methods are relatively rigorous and attempt to minimize personal bias. The researcher takes a logical approach and attempts to discover common patterns in a population. In nursing practice, however, skill is of paramount concern and methods are individualized. Clinical measures are relatively flexible, may rely on precedent, and call on clinical judgment. The clinician takes an intuitive approach and views each case as unique. These methodological differences are important because they affect the interactions that occur between the research and practice settings. Such differences have tended to preclude the use of research in practice as well as to inhibit the conduct of practice-relevant research. A process of methodological approximation, or a systematic effort to close the gap between research methods and practice methods, is essential to research utilization. Both researchers and clinicians need to assume responsibility for approximating one another's methods. The innovation protocol may be viewed as one step in a series of methodological approximations that are necessary for utilization. Later approximations can occur when nurses in a practice setting transform the protocol for their own particular needs and again when the change is implemented. The process used to develop innovation protocols will demonstrate this notion of methodological approximation.

The approach used to identify research-based knowledge with potential for use in nursing practice is based on the idea that there are areas of research in which studies can be related to one another by common variables and by relationships between those variables. Studies contributing to a particular area of research form the base from which nursing knowledge and nursing activities may be derived. When the activity suggested by the research base is different from traditional practice, that is, it either adds to practice in some way or calls for the extinction of a practice, it is an "innovation." Innovations in nursing imply changes in practice that are new to those using them and that are intended to benefit clients. Once a potential practice innovation has been identified, an attempt is made to "package" the information into an "innovation protocol"; this represents a methodological approximation of research to practice. An effort is made to write the protocols in a form that will be useful to nurses interested in implementing research-based planned change in nursing practice An innovation protocol, therefore, is research-based knowledge put in the form of a product; the product is nursing knowledge that has clearly definable parameters for use in practice.

THE PROTOCOL

At this point it might be useful to describe the form and content of an innovation protocol. Each protocol begins with a section on the need for change, documenting the extent of the clinical problem and the relevance of the problem to nursing practice. The second section gives a description of the innovation, including information on the types of patients most likely to benefit from the innovation. The protocol then provides a summary of the research base and identifies "research-based principles" to guide the implementation of the innovation. Although the use of the term "principle" is not scientifically accurate, CURN Project staff have persisted in using the term because it was found to communicate the appropriate intent to nurses who use the protocols. It is more accurate, however, to say that what are extracted from the research bases are empirical generalizations.

The remainder of the protocol deals with implementation of the innovation and systematic evaluation of its effects. With regard to both of these processes, the protocol describes the materials that will be required, the personnel development that may be necessary to carry out the activities suggested, and the costs that are likely to be incurred. Finally, each protocol is summarized by a discussion of the benefits that can be expected to result from a successful trial of the innovation. Additional materials may be appended to the protocols as they are available or can be developed. These materials always include the primary sources of the research base. They may also include an annotated bibliography, an evaluation procedure designed by the author of the protocol, and any additional tools or resources that are available from the original researchers.

Ten research-based practice protocols have been developed by project personnel and are being field tested. These include:

1. Structured preoperative teaching
2. A lactose-free diet
3. Sensation information: distress reduction
4. Sensory information: recovery rate
5. Nonsterile intermittent urinary catheterization
6. Prevention of catheter-associated urinary tract infections
7. Intravenous cannula change regimen
8. Prevention of decubiti by means of small shifts of body weight
9. Mutual goal setting: goal attainment
10. Deliberative nursing: pain reduction

CRITERIA FOR UTILIZATION OF RESEARCH IN NURSING PRACTICE

When project staff began the search and retrieval process for research bases, a number of well-known nursing researchers were asked to identify areas of clinical research which they felt were sufficiently developed to merit use in practice. Responses indicated a wide range of opinion; for example, some felt that "anything may be utilized; the determination rests with those who want to incorporate the ideas in any given study into their clinical work." Others responded toward the opposite end of the continuum: "No area of clinical nursing research is currently adequate for utilization in practice." Clearly such a range of answers suggested that different processes, criteria, and issues were considered by the respondents. The nursing literature also offered little assistance in defining how or with what criteria one may determine the adequacy of clinical research bases. Therefore, CURN Project personnel established criteria for selecting the research that is used in the development of protocols and in the utilization efforts of the project. The criteria were organized into three major categories: (a) criteria that pertain to evaluating and integrating studies that constitute a base, (b) criteria that address the issue of how relevant the base is for nursing practice, and (c) criteria related to the potential for evaluation in the clinical setting. Each of these will be discussed.

Evaluation and Integration of Studies

REPLICATION. The first criterion for identifying studies that constitute a research base is replication. Ideally there is more than one study in a research base to provide greater assurance against committing a Type I error, thereby inferring an effect where none exists. Some researchers criticize this approach by noting that the Type II error can be just as costly in inferring a lack of effect when there actually is one. Certainly, postponing implementation of a valid study is of concern; however, the possibility of implementing an innovation based on a "false positive" has legal and ethical ramifications that project personnel were unwilling to risk. Therefore, when developing protocols in any given area of research, an effort is made to establish that the conceptual and constructive propositions have been confirmed in more than one study; this is a process of construct replication. According to Lykken (1968), construct replication tests the validity of the "relation between meaningful constructs, generalizable to some broad reference population, which the [original author] claimed to have established" (p. 156). Construct replication is achieved when a second investigator begins with a similar problem statement but formulates original methods of measurement and design to verify the first author's findings. The advantage of construct replication over literal or operational replication is that it validates previous work, extends the findings, and offers great utility because it builds knowledge efficiently.

In order to obtain a solid research base for an innovation, it has been necessary to organize studies according to the concepts tested and to actively seek instances of construct replication. For example, numerous investigators (Felton, Huss, Payne, & Srsic, 1976; Fortin & Kirouac, 1976; Johnson, Rice, & Endress, 1975; Lindeman & Van Aernam, 1971) studied structured preoperative teaching and its postoperative effects. At the time the literature search was done, it was clear that these studies did not directly replicate one another. Yet the studies did demonstrate—in varied settings, using different populations, and a number of methodologies—that structured preoperative teaching does have a positive postoperative effect on clients. In other instances such replication has not been found. For example, numerous investigators studied various treatment modalities for decubitus ulcers (for a review of the literature, see Berecek, 1975). In these studies, to date, the findings are not corroborated: therefore, in spite of the extensiveness of the research, no base is available from which to develop a particular nursing innovation for treating decubitus ulcers.

SCIENTIFIC MERIT. The second criterion for studies constituting a research base is scientific merit. Each study with potential for contributing to the base is reviewed in terms of its design and methodology. Validity and reliability are key issues. The appropriateness of the sample for the clinical problem is also considered; generalizability is at issue here. At least one study in the research base must be conducted in a practice setting. Finally, the study's assumptions, findings, and conclusions are examined. The value of a study to the conceptual base is not determined entirely by the statistical significance of the findings; rather, an attempt is made to understand the functional relationships between variables in a base. The conclusions and implications of each study are evaluated in terms of their power to corroborate, extend, or delineate the conceptual base.

In the process of evaluating individual studies and comparing each with other studies in the base, conflicting findings may be found. Attempts are made to resolve contradictory findings either through identification of methodological weakness or through a theoretical explanation for the discrepancy. It is also recognized that in a series of replications of the same study, a nonsignificant difference may be expected to occur a certain number of times on the basis of chance alone. For example, the research base underlying the regimen for changing intravenous cannula consists of some 20 studies (e. g., Collin, Collin, Constable, & Johnston, 1975: Thomas, Evers, & Racz, 1970). Collectively, these studies support the proposition that duration of cannulization is positively related to local venous infection and infusion phlebitis. The findings of one study (Crossley & Matsen, 1972), however, resulted in a departure from this generalization. Closer scrutiny revealed that only intravenous infusions of greater than 24 hours' duration were included in the calculations. In truncating the data at one end of the scale, the significant effect of time on the dependent variables of infection and phlebitis may have been lost. Theoretically, this suggested that the findings were not necessarily contradictory to the research base but that there was probably a maximum time beyond which duration of the intravenous infusion does not correlate significantly with complications. Further search and retrieval was indicated to confirm this suspicion and to define what the maximum time might be. The example demonstrates that each study in a conceptual area is evaluated on its own scientific merit as well as on its power to contribute to a research base for practice by corroboration or extension.

RISK. The third criterion used to identify clinical research bases is risk. The concept of risk is used to mediate the stringency with which the criteria of replication and scientific merit are applied. Where the risk to the client is small, a generalization is made more readily than in those instances where the risk is great. For instance, studies exist that can be grouped conceptually into an area; yet, considered together, these studies do not deal fully with the functional relationships among the variables. There may be some weaknesses in methodology; there may be conflicting findings; or perhaps the case for construct replication is not strong. If there is little potential harm to the client, the practice action suggested by the research base may be tentatively implemented *pending clinical evaluation.* Such is the case in the decubitus prevention protocol. The nursing innovation derived from the base calls for unscheduled small shifts of body weight in addition to routine, scheduled turning. Although this research base has some weaknesses, implementation of the innovation requires little time or training on the part of the staff and does not jeopardize the client in any way. In other protocols where risk to the client is greater, the criteria have been applied more stringently.

Relevance to Practice

Once it has been established that a research base exists, the second major category of criteria needs to be considered; these criteria deal with the issue of practice relevance. When applied to an innovation, practice relevance means that the innovation derived from the base meets the demand of a nursing problem in a clinical setting. To state it another way, a research-based innovation that is practice relevant means that it has approximated the practice setting's goals and methods. The degree to which this approximation has occurred may be judged by four criteria: (a) degree of clinical merit, (b) extent of clinical control over the variables, (c) feasibility, and (d) cost.

CLINICAL MERIT. Clinical merit is the degree to which the research base addresses a problem of significance to the practice setting or the degree to which the suggested innovation will be potentially useful. Clinical merit represents an approximation of the research problem to the clinical goal.

CLINICAL CONTROL. A second consideration is clinical control. It is essential that nursing has, or is able to achieve, clinical control of the independent and dependent variables in the research base. If nurses are to use the research base, they must be in control of the events required for implementation and evaluation of the innovation. Control is problematic for two reasons: (a) the outcomes of nursing practice are often influenced by multiple factors external to the nurse–patient relationship; and (b) the instruments used to measure the effects of the innovation may not be available for use by nurses in the practice setting.

In the first instance, control over the outcomes of nursing practice is the concern. Occasionally, the variables in the research base fall clearly within the purview of nursing and control becomes almost automatic. An example of this occurs in the decubitus prevention protocol where the independent variable is small shifts of body weight and the dependent variable is occurrence of pressure sores. Clearly both variables are within the purview of nursing with minimal input from other professionals. In most of the protocols, however, clinical control of the variables must be achieved through the development of collaborative decision making with other practitioners. For instance, implementation of the nonsterile intermittent catheterization protocol requires cooperation with physicians. Input by physicians is necessary in making the decision to use nonsterile intermittent catheterization with individual patients, in prescribing drugs used in conjunction with the innovation, and in ordering laboratory studies to determine the effectiveness of the innovation. Clearly, securing the involvement of physicians is crucial to clinical control over implementation and evaluation of this innovation.

The second control problem relates to measurement. The protocols require the use of some of the dependent variables from the research base for evaluation of the innovation. Frequently, however, the methods that the researchers used to measure the dependent variables are not immediately available in the clinical setting. In some cases, an approximation to practice can be made by the substitution of valid clinical measures for the research instruments.

In other cases, the clinical setting may approximate the researchers' methods by acquiring the new knowledge or skill needed to use the research tools. When the preoperative teaching protocol was implemented in two different Michigan hospitals, one setting chose to substitute tape measurement of chest expansion and auscultation for spirometry as measures of respiratory status. This particular substitution was adapted from work done by Horn and Swain (1977) and demonstrates an approximation to practice. The second setting chose to work with the respiratory therapy department to gain access to the knowledge and skills needed to do spirometry; in this case, a clinical approximation to research methodology was made.

FEASIBILITY. Feasibility is the next factor that is considered in determining practice relevance. Given the constraints of the environments in which nurses practice, is it feasible to implement the innovation? Feasibility varies from institution to institution because it is related to the availability of resources (e.g., time, personnel, expertise, and equipment) and to the dominant feeling about change in the clinical setting. Each of these factors will vary in turn by the nature of the innovation, such as the degree of change it implies, the relative compatibility of the innovation with current nursing practice, the number of clients who will be affected, or the number of staff nurses to be involved.

COST BENEFITS. Closely related to feasibility but treated as a separate factor is cost. The financial cost of implementing and evaluating the innovation suggested by the research base is balanced against the potential benefit to clients. Since this type of analysis is rarely documented in the research literature, an estimate is made. Estimates most frequently balance the costs of materials, laboratory expenses, personnel development and staff time against such benefits as reduced incidence of complications and patient or staff satisfaction.

Potential for Clinical Evaluation

Each research base must be reviewed in relation to its potential for permitting adequate clinical evaluation of the proposed practice change. A key distinction between research utilization and replication of research points to the importance of clinical evaluation. Utilization implies that the practitioner transforms the new knowledge for use in the practice setting. Even under ideal conditions of clinical control, utilization of research in the clinical setting constitutes a change in the independent variable. To assure that this change or transformation has not extended beyond the limits of the research base, it must be possible to evaluate clinically the effects of the innovation once the protocol has been implemented. More specifically, the criterion states that there must be one or more dependent variables in the original research base that can be reliably measured by clinicians in practice settings. There are actually two components to this criterion: (a) the clinical knowledge and skills of the general nursing staff necessary to measure reliably the dependent variable and (b) the clinical control of the variable, which was discussed earlier. Using this criterion, project staff found that many of the dependent measures in the research base are not useful for clinical evaluation. Further, those measures that do meet the demands of the criterion are often the weakest in the research base in terms of validity and reliability.

PURPOSES OF INNOVATION EVALUATION. Evaluation of an innovation serves multiple purposes. Clinical evaluation moves practitioners to approximate research methodology more closely since such evaluation requires a systematic and controlled process involving measurement, data collection, and analysis. Evaluation can also be used to assess the extent to which research knowledge is applicable to practice settings. This information can then provide useful feedback to the original researchers. In addition, clinical evaluation questions whether the innovation is relevant to a practice problem, that is, whether or not it produces an outcome that justifies its use. The data base provided by clinical evaluation can serve to justify the new practice to others and is useful in meeting legal and ethical concerns related to accountability.

CHARACTERISTICS OF INNOVATION EVALUATION. Initially, it was anticipated that the research base would identify the outcome variables and also assist in the development of appropriate measurement procedures for use in evaluation. This has not always been true, and as a result greater flexibility has been required in the design of evaluation procedures to accompany the innovation. For instance, the original work on nonsterile intermittent catheterization was done by physicians. Some of the dependent variables, such as cystoscopy results, were not felt to be appropriate as nursing outcomes. On the other hand, some of the variables of keen interest to nursing were not accounted for in the research base; these included patient satisfaction, patient mobility, and degree of social interaction. Therefore, an evaluation procedure was devised that included variables from the research base and also drew on introspection about clinical practice.

Evaluation of the innovation is structured into a process component and an outcome component, providing a format that parallels current efforts in quality assurance. Independent variables from the research base are measured in terms of process to assure that the innovation has been implemented accurately and consistently; dependent variables are measured as outcomes. Once such an evaluation has been designed, it is easily placed into the ongoing quality assurance system.

To date, all evaluations use a pre- and postimplementation design. Baseline data and postimplementation data are usually summarized by frequency tables, ranges, rates, or means for purposes of comparison. Differences in the data are not tested for statistical significance. Again, a process of clinical evaluation rather than replication is advocated.

CONCLUSION

Development of research-based practice innovation protocols begins with a search for conceptually related studies that have potential for utilization in clinical nursing settings. Each potential practice area is then appraised according to the three major criteria that have been established by the CURN Project staff. If the area has an established research base, is practice relevant, and can be reliably evaluated by clinicians, it is judged sufficient for utilization in practice settings. An innovation protocol is subsequently developed, serving as a form of methodological approximation.

In many instances, potential practice innovations fail to meet the criteria and thus do not merit utilization in practice. Perhaps a replication of the original study is all that is necessary to permit its utilization, or it may be that a more valid and/or reliable tool is required in order to evaluate clinically the effects of the innovation. Through the process of subjecting each area to the demands of the criteria, missing links and deficiencies that preclude utilization become apparent. The identified deficiencies are of major importance, for they point to areas that need further research. Therefore, the process can also serve to guide future research efforts in nursing.

REFERENCES

Aydelotte, M. K. Nursing research in clinical settings: Problems and issues. *Sigma Theta Tau Reflections,* 1976, *2,* 3–6.

Berecek, K. H. Treatment of decubitus ulcers. *Nursing Clinics of North America,* 1975, *10,* 171–210.

Collin, J., Collin, C., Constable, F. L., & Johnston, I. D. A. Infusion thrombophlebitis and infection with various cannulas. *Lancet,* 1975, *2,* 150–153.

Crossley, K., & Matsen, J. M. The scalp-vein needle: A prospective study of complications. *Journal of the American Medical Association.* 1972, *220,* 985–987.

Felton, G., Huss, K., Payne, E. A., & Srsic, K. Preoperative nursing intervention with the patient for surgery: Outcomes of three alternative approaches. *International Journal of Nursing Studies,* 1976, *13,* 83–96.

Fortin, F., & Kirouac, S. A randomized controlled trial of preoperative patient education. *International Journal of Nursing Studies,* 1976, *13,* 11–24.

Horn, B. J., & Swain, M. A. Development of criterion measures of nursing care. Unpublished manuscript, School of Public Health, University of Michigan, 1977.

Horsley, J. A., Crane J., & Bingle, J. D. Research utilization as an organizational process. *Journal of Nursing Administration,* 1978, *8* (7), 4–6.

Johnson, J. E., Rice, V. H., & Endress, M. P. Making psychological concepts concrete for medical education. *Proceedings of the 14th Annual Conference on Research in Medical Education.* Washington, D.C.: Association of American Medical Colleges, 1975, 125–130.

Ketefian, S. Application of selected nursing research findings into nursing practice. *Nursing Research,* 1975, *24,* 89–92.

Krueger, J. C. Utilization of nursing research: The planning process. *Journal of Nursing Administration,* 1978, *8*(1), 6–9.

Lindeman, C. A., & Van Aernam, B. Nursing intervention with the presurgical patient—The effects of structured and unstructured preoperative teaching. *Nursing Research,* 1971, *20,* 319–332.

Lykken, D. T. Statistical significance in psychological research. *Psychological Bulletin,* 1968, *70,* 151–159.

Thomas, E. T., Evers, W., & Racz, G. B. Postinfusion phlebitis. *Anesthesia and Analgesia,* 1970, *49,* 150–159.

BIBLIOGRAPHY

Bayless, T. M., & Rosensweig, N. S. A racial difference in incidence of lactase deficiency. *Journal of the American Medical Association*, 1966, *197*, 138–142.

Bayless, T. M., Rothfeld, B., Massa, C., Wise, L., Paige, D., & Bedine, M. S. Lactose and milk intolerance: Clinical implications. *The New England Journal of Medicine*, 1975, *292*, 1156–1159.

Bedine, M. S., & Bayless, M.D. Intolerance of small amounts of lactose by individuals with low lactase levels. *Gastroenterology*, 1973, *65*, 735–743.

Gault, M. H., Dixon, M. E., Doyle, M., & Cohen, W. M. Hypernatremia, azotemia, and dehydration due to high-protein tube feeding. Annals of Internal Medicine, 1968, *68*, 778–791.

Haller, K. B., Reynolds, M. A., & Horsley, J. A. Developing research-based innovation protocols: Process, criteria, and issues. *Research in Nursing and Health,* 1979, *2,* 45–51.

Hanson, R. L., Walike, B. C., Grant, M., Kubo, W., Bergstrom, N., Padilla, G., & Wong, H. L. Patient responses and problems associated with tube feeding. *Washington State Journal of Nursing,* Winter 1975, pp. 9–13.

Horsley, J. A., Crane, J., & Bingle, J. D. Research utilization as an organizational process. *Journal of Nursing Administration,* 1978, *8* (7), 4–6.

Johnson, J. D., Kretchmer, N., & Simoons, F. J. Lactose malabsorption: Its biology and history. *Advances in Pediatrics,* 1974, *21,* 197–237.

Jones, E. S. & Peaston, M.J.T. Metabolic care during acute illnesses. *The Practitioner,* 1966, *196,* 271–275.

Kubo, W., Grant, M., Walike, B., Bergstrom, N., Wong, H., Hanson, R., & Padilla, G. Fluid and electrolyte problems of tube-fed patients. *American Journal of Nursing,* 1976, *76,* 912–916.

Lysaught, J. P. *Abstract for action.* New York: McGraw-Hill Book Co., 1970.

Minckley, B. B. Critique of "patient problems related to tube feeding." In M. V. Batey (Ed.), *Communicating Nursing Research* (vol. 7). Boulder, Colo.: WICHE, 1975.

Pareira, M. D. *Therapeutic nutrition with tube feeding.* Springfield, Ill.: Chas. C Thomas, 1959.

Rosenberg, F. H. Lactose intolerance. *American Journal of Nursing,* 1977, *77,* 823–824.

Walike, B. C. Disturbances of food intake and nutrition. In H. Moidel, B. Wagner, and E. Giblin (Eds.), *Nursing care of the patient with medical–surgical disorders* (2nd ed.). New York: McGraw-Hill Co., 1976.

Walike, B. C., Padilla, G., Bergstrom, N., Hanson, R. L., Kubo, W., Grant, M., & Wong, H. L. Patient problems related to tube feeding. In M. V. Batey (Ed.), *Communicating Nursing Research* (vol. 7). Boulder, Colo.: WICHE, 1975.

Walike, B. C., & Walike, J. W. Lactose content of tube feeding diets as a cause of diarrhea. *The Laryngoscope,* 1973, *83,* 1109–1115.

Walike, B. C., & Walike, J. W. Relative lactose intolerance. *Journal of the American Medical Association,* 1977, *238,* 948–951.

Walike, B. C., Walike, J. W., Hanson, R. L., Grant, M., Kubo, W., Bergstrom, N. Wong, H. L., Padilla, G., & Williams, K. Nasogastric tube feeding: Clinical complications and current progress of research. *Northwest Health Team Approach,* 1975, *2,* (6), 33–41.

Walike, J. W. Tube-feeding syndrome in head and neck surgery. *Archives of Otolaryngology,* 1969, *89,* 533–536.

Welsh, J. D. Isolated lactase deficiency in humans: Report on 100 patients. *Medicine,* 1970, *49,* 257–277.

INDEX